D. P. LANE
CRC GROUP
BIOCHEM DEPT
IMPERIAL COLLEGE
LONDON SW7 2AZ

ADVANCES IN VIRAL ONCOLOGY

Volume 2

*The Transformation-Associated
Cellular p53 Protein*

Advances in Viral Oncology

Volume 2

The Transformation-Associated Cellular p53 Protein

Editor

George Klein, M.D., D.Sc.
Department of Tumor Biology
Karolinska Institutet
Stockholm, Sweden

Raven Press ∎ New York

Raven Press, 1140 Avenue of the Americas, New York, New York 10036

Library of Congress Cataloging in Publication Data
Main entry under title:

The Transformation-associated cellular p53 protein.

    (Advances in viral oncology ; v. 2)
    Includes bibliographical references and index.
    Contents: The origins of p53 in relation to
transformation / Lionel Crawford -- The complex
between p53 and SV40 T antigen / D.P. Lane,
J. Gannon, and G. Winchester -- Monoclonal antibody
analysis of a cellular tumor antigen / Elizabeth G.
Gurney -- [etc.]
    1. Carcinogenesis. 2. Viral carcinogenesis.
3. Simian vacuolating virus. 4. Proteins.
I. Klein, George, 1925-   II. Series.
III. Title: p53 protein.   [DNLM: 1. Cell transformation, Neoplastic. 2. Cell transformation, Viral.
3. Neoplasm proteins. W1 AD888 v.2 / QZ 200 T772]
RC268.5.T68   1982   616.99'4071   82-11209
ISBN 0-89004-857-6

Made in the United States of America

Preface

This volume focuses on recent evidence concerned with the discovery and the transformation-related role of 53–55K cellular protein, expressed by the many forms of RNA and DNA virus-induced tumors as well as by tumors of nonviral origin. The switch-on of this protein may form a link between the very different fields of RNA and DNA virus-mediated transformation.

In dealing with this topic, we have tried to bring together a representative assembly of the primary authors responsible for the development in this field. In view of the multiple approach toward the common target, a certain overlapping could not be avoided and was actually considered desirable. This topic provides a bridge toward a later volume that will deal with the transforming action of the DNA tumor viruses.

This volume is written for the specialist in cancer research and/or viral oncology who wishes to be informed about the recent developments in this area.

George Klein

Introduction—Nomenclature

Because of the way in which work on p53 developed in a large variety of different systems many different terms have been used for what now appears to be the same group of proteins. Terms such as "SV40 middle-T," "56K," "55K," "54K," "53K," "p53," "p50," "48K," "NVT," and "Tau" have all been used by various groups. None of these terms is entirely satisfactory and, indeed, "SV40 middle-T" is distinctly misleading.

Nevertheless, the contributors to this volume have all agreed for the sake of uniformity to use "p53" here in preference to other names. The name is to some extent arbitrary and will clearly be superceded when the function of p53 is defined and a corresponding functional name devised. The protein referred to as p53 is heterogeneous on two-dimensional gels in a given species and has different mobilities in different species. Its properties will be defined in the articles which follow and the reasons for our assumption that it is indeed the same, or equivalent, in each context, will then be clearer.

Lionel Crawford

Contents

Contributors

Ettore Appella. *Laboratory of Cell Biology, National Cancer Institute, National Institutes of Health, Bethesda, Maryland 20205*

Andrea A. Blum. *Department of Pathology, New York University Medical School, New York, New York 10016*

Robert B. Carroll. *Department of Pathology, New York University Medical School, New York, New York 10016*

Lionel Crawford. *Molecular Virology Laboratory, Imperial Cancer Research Fund, London WC2A 3PX, England*

J. Gannon. *Cancer Research Campaign, Eukaryotic Molecular Genetics Research Group, Department of Biochemistry, Imperial College, London SW7, England*

Daniel S. Greenspan. *Department of Pathology, New York University Medical School, New York, New York 10016*

Elizabeth G. Gurney. *Department of Biology, University of Utah, Salt Lake City, Utah 84112*

Vincent J. Hearing. *Dermatology Branch, National Cancer Institute, National Institutes of Health, Bethesda, Maryland 20205*

Hans Jörnvall. *Department of Chemistry I, Karolinska Institutet, S-104 01 Stockholm, Sweden*

Michel Kress. *Institute for Cancer Research, 94802 Villejuif Cedex, France*

D. P. Lane. *Cancer Research Campaign, Eukaryotic Molecular Genetics Research Group, Department of Biochemistry, Imperial College, London SW7, England*

A. J. Levine. *State University of New York at Stony Brook, Department of Microbiology, School of Medicine, Stony Brook, New York 11794*

Janos Luka. *Department of Tumor Biology, Karolinska Institutet, S-104 01 Stockholm, Sweden*

Evelyne May. *Institute for Cancer Research, 94802 Villejuif Cedex, France*

Pierre May. *Institute for Cancer Research, 94802 Villejuif Cedex, France*

M. Oren. *State University of New York at Stony Brook, Department of Microbiology, School of Medicine, Stony Brook, New York 11794*

N. Reich. *State University of New York at Stony Brook, Department of Microbiology, School of Medicine, Stony Brook, New York 11794*

P. Sarnow. *State University of New York at Stony Brook, Department of Microbiology, School of Medicine, Stony Brook, New York 11794*

G. Winchester. *Cancer Research Campaign, Eukaryotic Molecular Genetics Research Group, Department of Biochemistry, Imperial College, London SW7, England*

The Transformation-Associated Cellular p53 Protein

Advances in Viral Oncology, Volume 2, edited by
George Klein. Raven Press, New York © 1982.

The Origins of p53 in Relation to Transformation

Lionel Crawford

*Molecular Virology Laboratory, Imperial Cancer Research Fund,
Lincoln's Inn Fields, London WC2A 3PX, England*

In viruses such as SV40 where infection does not suppress the synthesis of host proteins, it has always been difficult to decipher the virus-specific changes from the predominant background of host-specific protein synthesis. This is even more difficult in transformed cells where the contribution of virus-specific protein synthesis may be less than 1% of the total. One solution to this problem of discrimination between virus-related proteins and the rest has proved to be through the application of immunological techniques. Initially these were relatively crude, relying as they did on sera from tumor-bearing animals as source of specific antibodies. Despite the limitations inherent in the methods, they produced very significant advances in the detection and characterization of virus-specific products in transformed cells and in defining their relationship to the transformed state. Subsequent advances have come largely from application of improved immunological techniques in the first step with antisera of defined specificity rather than the antisera from tumor-bearing animals with their wider but less well-defined specificity. The second step in this direction of increasing definition of antibody came with isolation of hybridomas producing monoclonal antibodies, each recognizing a specific determinant on the several antigens involved, and opening the way for application of a great variety of sophisticated methods for the separation and quantitation of these antigens. At the same time, and equally important technically, was the change from double antibody immunoprecipitation to the use of protein A-Staphylococci as immunoadsorbent. This was particularly important in studies of p53 and other antigens in the 50,000 to 60,000 molecular weight range since excessive amounts of immunoglobulin heavy chain on polyacrylamide gels distorted and obscured this region very badly. All these improvements in immunological techniques went hand in hand with the rapidly advancing understanding of the molecular biology of SV40 and related viruses. The determination of the nucleotide sequence of SV40 (14,28) provided the foundation for understanding the way in which the virus-coded antigens were related to each other and distinct from the host-coded ones.

VIRUS-CODED ANTIGENS

The first virus-coded antigen to be defined for SV40 was the product of the A cistron, large-T, with an apparent molecular weight of 94,000 (30). Since this protein seemed to take up virtually the entire coding capacity of the early region of the virus, it was difficult to see how any other protein could be coded within this region of the virus genome. This seemed, therefore, to be the total virus-coded contribution to transformed cells in which only the early region was expressed. Other proteins precipitable with anti-tumor sera had already been observed in *in vitro* protein synthesizing systems, but the corresponding proteins were not observed reproducibly in extracts of transformed or infected cells for reasons that are clearer now than they were at the time. By bringing together variable deletion mutants, *in vitro* protein synthesis, and improved immunoprecipitation techniques with the idea of RNA splicing, it was possible to construct a coherent explanation of how small-t could be coded within the region of the virus genome, already known to code for large-T (7). Since a single region of the genome could code for two proteins with splices occurring within the protein-coding sequence, there was no reason why a third protein could not be accommodated. In the case of polyoma virus, the coding region for a third protein, middle-T (18,19), was in fact so located but the defined nucleotide sequence of SV40 made it very difficult to see how such a third protein could be coded within its early region without invoking very ornate splicing patterns.

HOST-CODED TUMOR ANTIGENS

Proteins of about the same size as polyoma middle-T had been observed in immunoprecipitates in the earliest studies of infected and transformed cells (32) and many times subsequently. These proteins must have included p53, but other material may also have contributed bands to the same region of the gels. Proteolytic cleavage of large-T certainly occurred with the extraction procedures then in use. Although this was more marked with infected than with transformed cells and gave rise to the idea that large-T was smaller in infected than transformed cells (1,4), it made interpretation of these observations difficult. One particular band of 60,000 molecular weight was, for example, shown to be closely related to large-T, retaining its reactivity with anti-T polypeptide serum (11). Other bands in the intermediate size range of gels from immunoprecipitated cell extracts included host proteins, such as actin and tubulin, which tend to precipitate due to polymerization. In the presence of immune complexes, this precipitation is accentuated. Thus, material in the region of p53 included this protein but its contribution to the total protein was variable and it could, in some circumstances, be only a small fraction of the total.

Throughout the studies of p53 in SV40-transformed cells, at this stage, there was the difficulty of reconciling two conflicting sets of data. Although p53 seemed to be virus-specific, its size and tryptic peptide patterns were markedly dependent on the host cell. This gave rise to the idea of hybrid messenger RNAs derived in part from the integrated virus DNA and in part from the host cell DNA, either adjacent to the integrated DNA or perhaps even drawn from distant sequences by splicing between different initial transcripts. This type of model would predict that amino acid sequences common to known virus-coded antigens would probably appear in p53 if the same reading frame were used in translation of the common regions in the two cases. This could lead to immunological cross-reaction between large-T and p53. Such a cross-reaction was reported (3,26), although it was too weak to have provided an entirely satisfactory explanation for the precipitation of p53 normally observed in extracts of SV40-transformed cells. It now seems likely that there is no major cross-reaction between p53 and SV40 large-T. Cross-reactions between host proteins and large-T have been observed with several monoclonal antibodies recently (9,21). Only a few of the anti-T monoclonal antibodies so far examined (16) show this type of cross-reaction and, as yet, there is no instance in which p53 is the host protein involved.

THE COMPLEX OF p53 AND LARGE-T

The resolution of this problem of reconciling the virus-specific but host-influenced nature of p53 came from the demonstration that in transformed cells p53 was associated in a specific and stable complex with SV40 large-T and that its precipitation was in most cases due to this association (20). Specific antiserum prepared against gel-purified large-T (20) was critical for this demonstration and, since it retained activity against denatured polypeptides, could be used in direct radioimmunoassays to distinguish those proteins that had reactivity in their own right and p53, which had lacked such reactivity but could coprecipitate with large-T. The same specific anti-denatured polypeptide serum that precipitated p53 coordinately with large-T in cell extracts lacked activity against the denatured p53 polypeptide in the absence of large-T. Complementary studies with a rabbit anti-p53 serum (25) completed the proof of the existence of the SV40 large-T antigen-p53 complex and facilitated estimation of the amounts of free and complexed large-T and p53. The direct radioimmunoassay (22) also allowed the detection of significant levels of anti-p53 activity in some anti-tumor sera (20). With this activity it could be shown that p53 was prominent not only in SV40-transformed cells but also in polyoma virus-transformed cells (8,20) and in teratocarcinoma cells where there was no virus involved at all (23). This showed clearly that p53 was a host-coded protein and that there was no longer any need to invoke any virus-coded contribution at all. The convergence of work on virus-transformed cells with that on cells transformed by chemical carcinogens (12) showed just how widespread the involvement of p53 with transformation of all types was, in contrast to the highly individual antigenic changes previously observed with tumors induced in different animals by different, or even the same, agent(s).

p53 IN HUMAN TUMOR CELL LINES

Once it had been established that changes in p53 were widespread among mouse cells transformed by different agents, then it was natural to ask whether the same was true of human tumor cells. This involved making use of both the techniques and reagents developed for the SV40-transformed mouse cell system. Although the anti-p53 activity of serum from tumor bearing mice against human p53 is low, some of the antibodies present must react with both mouse and human p53. Because both are host proteins, they are related but not identical, and seem to share about half their tryptic peptides (31). Fortunately, the first anti-p53 monoclonal antibody to be isolated was human/mouse cross-reactive (15) and could be used to answer this question. It was not clear at first whether human cells contained a protein equivalent to mouse p53 by the criterion of its ability to form a complex with SV40 large-T. Whether large-T and p53 coprecipitated depended to some extent on the way that the cell extracts were made and the conditions that were used for forming and washing the immunoprecipitates. As shown in Fig. 1, the normal extraction conditions leave most of the mouse p53 complexed with large-T, whereas a substantial fraction of human p53 appears free of the complex. This reflects the difference in stability between complexes of SV40 large-T with rodent p53 as compared to primate p53, the primate complex being less stable (17). In other ways the mouse and human p53 were very similar in the corresponding SV40-transformed cells, although differing significantly in their mobility on polyacrylamide gels. Mouse p53 can be separated by two-dimensional gels into a number of components in both

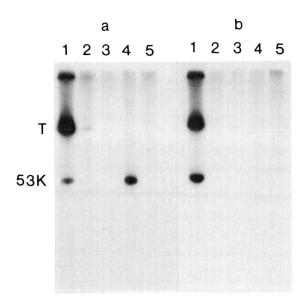

FIG. 1. Cascade immunoprecipitation of large T antigen and p53 from SV40-transformed cells. Extracts of ³²P-labeled human (*a*) and mouse *(b)* cells were treated sequentially with antisera as follows: track 1, anti-T serum D2 and SAC; track 2, same as track 1; track 3, SAC alone followed by either 4 or 5; track 4, anti-p53 antibody, PAb122, and SAC; track 5, same as track 1. After immunoprecipitation, the proteins were separated on a 12% polyacrylamide gel. (From Crawford et al., ref. 9.)

isoelectric focusing and SDS dimensions (8), indicating that it is a family of polypeptides rather than a single species. This is also true of human p53 from SV80 cells (Fig. 2). Two components with different mobilities in the SDS dimension both contain several species with different isoelectric points ranging between pH 6 and 7 with considerable streaking. Human p53 always moves more slowly than mouse p53 on SDS gels, but does not always show the doublet

FIG. 2. Isoelectric focusing of p53 from human tumor and SV40-transformed cells. Cell extracts were immunoprecipitated with PAb122 and the proteins were separated by the method of O'Farrell et al. (26). *a,* ³⁵S-Methionine-labeled SV80 cell extract. *b,* ³²P-phosphate-labeled SV80 cell extract. *c,d,e,* ³²P-phosphate-labeled extracts from human tumor cell lines; only the p53 region is shown, aligned so that regions of the same pI are vertically below each other and correspond to b. (From Crawford et al., ref. 9.)

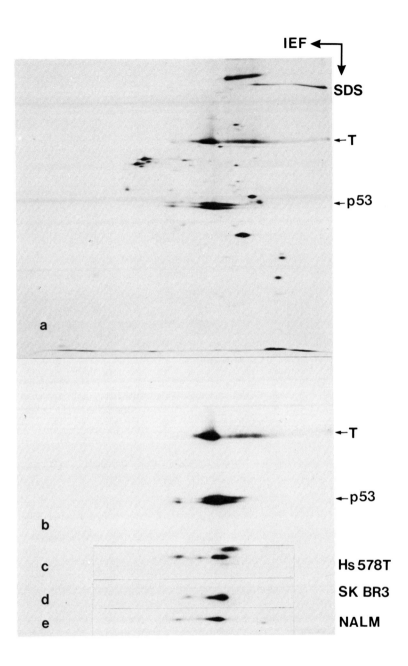

IEF

SDS

←T

←p53

a

←T

←p53

b

c   Hs 578T

d   SK BR3

e   NALM

seen with p53 from SV80 cells. Other human cell lines, derived from malignant tumors and not known to have any involvement of SV40, also show p53. This is very similar to p53 from SV80 cells in its behavior on two-dimensional gels (Fig. 2) and appears to be the equivalent protein by the following criteria. They are phospho-proteins, which react with monoclonal antibody PAb122 and have the same mobility on SDS gels and pI range on isoelectric focusing gels. In some cases at least, p53 forms a complex with SV40 large-T when the tumor cell lines are infected with SV40. The overall structures of the p53 proteins from tumor cell lines and from SV80 cells are also similar when compared by partial proteolysis (5), as shown in Fig. 3. In a survey of a variety of cell lines derived from tumors of epithelial and mesodermal origin, p53 was found in most but not all of the lines (Table 1) (10). Immunoprecipitation of p53 from ^{32}P-labeled cell extracts with anti-p53 monoclonal antibody (PAb122) was the test used. The difference in p53 labeling between normal human cells in culture and the tumor cell lines is quantitative rather than qualitative. Cultures of human foreskin fibroblast cells labeled with ^{35}S-methionine have subsequently been shown to give a very weak band of p53 that is authentic by the criterion of its partial proteolysis pattern (K. Leppard, *unpublished results*). The exceptional lines in which p53 could not be detected, such as HeLa, showed that rapid growth in culture was not by itself sufficient to accentuate p53, but they also raised the question of whether the methods used for detection of p53 were adequate or not. The lack of detectable p53 is not a peculiarity of cell lines derived from cervical carcinomas since another line examined later, C33-I (2), was positive and one line of bladder carcinoma cells, EJ, was neg-ative. All this depended heavily on the properties of a particular monoclonal antibody, PAb122, although other tests such as asso-ciation with SV40 large-T were used. Loss from p53 of the deter-minant recognized by PAb122 antibody would clearly generate a misleading false negative, in that the p53 in this case could be in other ways very similar to the reactive p53. For this reason we were eager to examine other anti-p53 monoclonal antibodies.

COMPARISON OF ANTI-p53 ANTIBODIES

Several anti-p53 antibodies are available now in addition to PAb122. These include PAb410 and PAb421 isolated by Ed Harlow. The hybridomas producing these antibodies were derived from mice bearing tumors of VLM (SV40-transformed) mouse cells and are similar in that respect to PAb122. Another antibody, PAb607, from a hybridoma isolated by Linda Gooding, also comes from this type of immunization. The other p53 antibodies come from other regimes—200.47 from mice bearing methylcholanthrene-induced tumors (13) and RA3 2C2 from mice bearing Abelson mouse leukemia virus-induced tumors (6,29). All of these anti-p53 monoclonal antibodies recognize determinants displayed on complexed mouse p53. This is shown by the fact that they precipitate both p53 and large-T from extracts of SV40 transformed mouse cells. In some cases they also have other activities. RA3 2C2 reacts with a differentiation specific antigen present on the surface of B lymphocytes (29) as discussed by Goff and Baltimore (*see Volume 1*). PAb410 and PAb421 cross-react with a 80,000 molecular weight protein in mouse cells, although this protein does not appear to be related to p53 in any obvious way (B. Kuypers, *unpublished results*). It is not a dimer of p53 nor is it associated with p53 and thus coprecipitated. These cross-reactions may be analogous to those already mentioned between large-T and host proteins. To make full use of these antibodies, we first wished to find out whether they reacted with the same determinants on p53 or, as we hoped, with different determinants. The availability of antibodies recognizing a range of determinants distributed over the molecule would extend the range of our methods for detecting and characterizing proteins related to mouse p53 in human tumor cells.

COMPETITION BETWEEN p53 ANTIBODIES

To elucidate the relationship between the determinants on p53 recognized by the various monoclonal antibodies, we have made

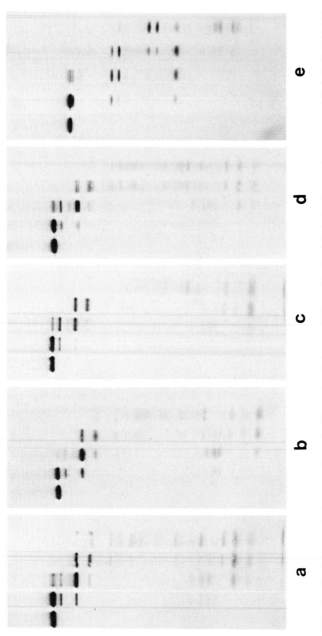

FIG. 3. Partial proteolysis comparison of p53 species. Extracts of ³⁵S-methionine-labeled cells were immunoprecipitated with PAb122 and the p53 were separated by gel electrophoresis. The gel bands were excised, and the polypeptides were digested with increasing amounts of *S. aureus* V8 protease for 1 hr at 37°C. The protease concentrations in each panel were, from left to right, 0, 0.2, 2, 20, and 200 μg/ml. The p53 species were derived from BT 20 (*a*), SV80 lower band (*b*), SV80 upper band (*c*), and Daudi (*d*). The 45,000-dalton band (*e*) was cut from the BT 20 gel and serves as a control. (From Crawford et al. ref. 9.)

TABLE 1. *The occurrence of p53 in human tumor cell lines and normal cell cultures[a]*

Cells	Type of tumor	p53
Lines		
Daudi	Burkitt lymphoma	+
Bristol 7	Lymphocyte transformed by EBV	+
NALM 1	Chronic myelogenous leukemia	+
BT 20	Primary mammary carcinoma	+
SK BR3	Metastatic mammary carcinoma	+
T47D	Metastatic mammary carcinoma	+
Hs 578T	Primary mammary carcinosarcoma	+
Tera 1	Teratocarcinoma	+
Tera 2	Teratocarcinoma	+
MG	Teratocarcinoma	+
BeWo	Choriocarcinoma	+
Jar	Choriocarcinoma	+
HeLa D98	Cervical carcinoma	−
C33I	Cervical carcinoma	+
EJ	Bladder carcinoma	−
Strains		
FS	Foreskin fibroblast culture	−
LN75	Skin fibroblast (Lesch-Nyhan)	−
Milk secondary culture	Mammary epithelium	−

[a]The origins of the cell lines are given in Crawford et al. (9), except for EJ, which was isolated by Dr. J. Daly (Massachusetts General Hospital) and is described in Marshall et al. (23).
The data are taken from Crawford et al. (9).

use of a solid state competition assay originally devised for a set of anti-T monoclonal antibodies. In this assay, one antibody is adsorbed to the wells of plastic microtiter plates and used to adsorb the antigen from a crude cell lysate. Other antibodies can then be used in competition with each other to bind to the fixed antigen. In each competition, one of the antibodies is labeled with ^{125}I so that blocking of the uptake of radioactivity onto the plate by the unlabeled antibodies, either of the same type or heterologous, can be followed (Fig. 4). One essential requirement is that the first antibody, the one used for binding the antigen to the plate, should react with the antigen independently of any of the antibodies under test, either ^{125}I labeled or unlabeled. To minimize any interference with the binding of any of the p53 antibodies in our preliminary assays, we took

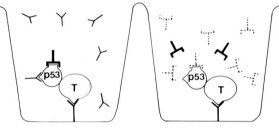

No competition   **Competition**

FIG. 4. Schematic representation of competition radioimmunoassay. PAb419 (anti-SV40 large-T antibody) was first adsorbed to the wells of PVC microtiter trays (1 μg of IgG per well in 50 μl of 10 mM phosphate buffer pH 7 overnight). The wells were then exposed to extracts of SV40-transformed mouse cells and the T-p53 complex adsorbed for 2 hr. The anti-p53 monoclonal antibodies were then allowed to compete for the available p53. In each case, one antibody was ^{125}I labeled and the competition of homologous and heterologous unlabeled antibodies compared with the result shown in Table 2. The radioactive antibody ⊥, the homologous non-radioactive antibody ⌐⌐, and the heterologous non-radioactive antibody ⋋ are shown.

advantage of the large-T-p53 complex from transformed mouse cells and used an anti-T monoclonal, PAb419 (16), as first antibody. This binds p53 via large-T and should block only the region of p53 involved in binding to large-T. The competition between PAb410, PAb421, and PAb122 showed that there was strong and reciprocal blocking between these antibodies in all combinations (Table 2). The relevant determinants are therefore close to or overlapping with each other. This is not surprising for PAb410 and PAb421, since they share many other properties with each other. They are the same IgG subclass, 2a, and both precipitate the 80,000 host protein from untransformed mouse cell extracts already mentioned. PAb122, on the other hand, is in a different subclass, IgG 2b, and can also be distinguished from PAb410 and PAb412 in that it does not react with the 80,000 protein. The determinants that are recognized by PAb410, PAb421, and PAb122 are therefore not identical but must be sufficiently close on the native p53 molecule that binding to one obscures the other. Incidentally, all three antibodies react with denaturation stable determinants and react equally well with primate and rodent p53 (15,16). Similar competition assays with RA3 2C2 and 200.47 showed that neither blocked the binding to ^{125}I-labeled

TABLE 2. *Competition between anti-p53 monoclonal antibodies[a]*

Competing antibody	Probe				
	PAb410	PAb421	PAb607	RA3 2C2	PAb122
PAb410	8	4	101	102	18
PAb421	6	6	90	88	10
PAb607	101	102	13	108	110
RA3 2C2	85	78	90	18	87
PAb122	14	9	80	85	18
200.47	97	90	100	100	92
Control	(100)	(100)	(100)	(100)	(100)

[a]Monoclonal antibody PAb419 was used to attach the SV40 large-T-p53 complex from an extract of SVA31E7 cells to PVC microtiter wells. The ^{125}I labeled antibodies were then allowed to compete with unlabeled antibody for the available p53 on the plastic. The figures shown are radioactively bound to the well as percent of the control (unrelated monoclonal antibody).

PAb421 to any great extent. This is the first indication that different determinants on p53 are being recognized by these various antibodies. It is not clear why p53 becomes antigenic in tumor-bearing animals despite its being a host protein. Possibly association with large-T causes an allosteric change in p53 that can then be recognized as foreign. The altered region might be close to the binding site and quite limited in extent so that most p53 antibodies would be directed toward a particular region of the molecule. This would not be the case with RA3 2C2 and 200.47, where SV40 was not involved in the immunization. In the case of RA3 2C2, it is not clear whether p53 was involved in the immunization at all or whether it is simply cross-reacting with the surface antigen of the B lymphocytes that acted as the immunogen.

Not all the anti-p53 monoclonal antibodies from SV40 tumor bearing mice are of the same type as PAb122, PAb410, and PAb421. PAb607, which comes from this type of immunization, is clearly different from PAb410 and PAb421. There was no significant blocking of PAb607 by PAb410 or PAb421 or vice versa (Table 2). It would seem, therefore, that there are at least four independent determinants on mouse p53. This gave us the opportunity of devising a radioimmunoassay for p53 from rodent cells.

With one of the anti-p53 antibodies attached to the microtiter plate, p53 could be adsorbed from the cell extract under test and then assayed by binding of a second p53 antibody. One of the beauties of this type of assay is that it is not affected by the fact that the various antibodies react with proteins other than p53. So long as the anti-p53 reactivity is the only element they share, the other activities will be irrelevant. Either the other protein will not be attached to the plastic in the second step or it will fail to pick up the antibody in the last step. The antibody pairs were selected on the basis of the data shown in Table 2. Preliminary results of this type of assay showed that there were high levels of p53 in SVA31E7 cells, moderate levels in 3T6 cells, and low levels in 3T3 A31 cells, as expected. We are currently using the assay to follow the effect of culture conditions on p53 levels in a variety of cell types.

DISCUSSION

In the last decade, tumor virology has been one of the most active and productive areas of cancer research. The molecular structures of the viruses as well as events in their life cycles, in both lytic and transforming interactions, have been elucidated in great detail, revealing a level of complexity and sophistication previously unsuspected and justifying the enormous amount of effort expended. With this knowledge we can now define the gene products of the various viruses that are implicated in the process of transformation, although in no case can a detailed explanation be given of the mechanisms by which the action of these gene products lead to the many phenotypic changes that distinguish transformed cells from the normal counterparts. Even so, it is clear that the mode of transformation is by no means always the same. Viruses as closely related as polyoma and SV40 differ, polyoma middle-T being implicated as the transforming protein of that virus and SV40 large-T as its transforming protein. For this reason, it is difficult to devise a unitary explanation for transformation, even if we restrict ourselves to the DNA viruses. In retrospect it may have been naive to expect the studies of DNA tumor viruses to be of direct help in understanding the sort of malignant transformation that leads to spontaneous tumors. DNA viruses always add genetic information to the transformed cell in the form of all, or part, of their early regions. Spontaneous transformation, on the other hand, seems more likely to result from rearrangement of genetic material than from addition of exogenous sequences. In this respect, RNA tumor viruses come closer to spontaneous transformation in that the gene for the transforming protein that they introduce is a cellular gene. Alternatively, they may alter the context and thus the control of the relevant cellular gene. In both cases the gene or a closely related one is already present in the cell before transformation. Even here it is not easy to see how the presence of an increased amount of a protein, such as a protein phosphokinase near the cell surface, actually results in transformation. Thus the great variety of mechanisms that seem to be used by the various DNA and RNA tumor viruses makes it difficult to extract from one such system elements relevant to understanding the others. If each transforming agent causes transformation by a quite separate pathway, then it is clear that little of what we learn from studying such systems will be of use in our efforts to understand the causation of spontaneous human tumors. As an alternative, we may envisage the chains of events in each of the different types of transformation as being initially separate, but progressively coming together to follow one, or a few, common pathways. From this common pathway, the different types may then branch out again to give rise to the many and varied phenotypic consequences of transformation. Which properties are shown may depend to a large extent on the type of cell involved and its physiology and location with respect to other cells.

The greater the common element in the pathway of transformation the better would be the prospect of understanding spontaneous transformation by analogy with experimental systems of *in vitro* transformation. The realization that the metabolism of p53 was altered in a great variety of transformed mouse cells raised the possibility that p53 might be part of just such a common pathway of transformation. There is, of course, one strong reservation in that laboratory mouse strains and *in vitro* transformation of their cells are not the same thing as the *in vivo* transformation by which human tumors are initiated. As a first step to meeting this sort of reservation we made use of the technology and reagents developed in studies of SV40 transformation of mouse cells to look at human tumor cell lines *in vitro*. It was very encouraging to find that in many such lines there was a clear increase in the prominence of p53. Having verified that the situation was thus similar to that in the transformed mouse cells, the next step was to move closer to the tumors themselves. Human tumor cell lines may not be very representative of tumors *in vivo* for two reasons: First, many tumors, especially, it seems, highly malignant ones, do not easily give rise to cell lines *in vitro*, and second, there is no guarantee that the cells that grow out of the minority of tumors that do grow *in vitro* are the same cells that were growing malignantly *in vivo*. To answer questions about the status of p53 *in vivo* requires assays for the amount of the protein in tissue samples and some means of studying the control of its synthesis, messenger RNA levels and so on. A start has been made on the protein assay requirement by making use of the remarkable properties of monoclonal antibodies, and parallel advances with cloning of the gene for p53 should facilitate studies on the control of its synthesis. To carry out a comprehensive study of p53 in tumors will necessitate a great deal of work, and it would be nice to have some indication that p53 really is involved in human tumors. The evidence that we have is both indirect and preliminary, but it does implicate p53. Although p53 is a host protein, it is possible for it to be rendered immunogenic in transformed cells, perhaps by some change in amount, location, or allosteric configuration. The isolation of hybridomas, which produce anti-p53 monoclonal antibodies from mice carrying tumors of SV40-transformed or methylcholanthrene-transformed cells, shows that this can occur with or without the involvement of a virus-coded protein such as large-T, which complexes with p53. If cancer patients were found to have circulating anti-p53 antibodies, this would perhaps be an indication that the alteration of p53 metabolism in spontaneous tumors was similar in that it rendered p53 immunogenic. In our initial survey of a small number of patients suffering from mammary carcinomas (L. Crawford and R. D. Bulbrook, *unpublished results*), what appeared to be anti-p53 activity was detected in the sera of a minority of patients who had suffered recurrence of tumors after surgical removal of the primary tumor. Sera from normal women showed no detectable activity. It should be emphasized that the number of patients studied is still very small, and it is possible that a more extended study will show that there is no significant increase in anti-p53 antibodies in other cancer patients. We are sufficiently encouraged, however, to continue with these studies and with the idea that p53 is involved in some significant way with human tumors.

ACKNOWLEDGMENTS

I would like to thank my colleagues at the Imperial Cancer Research Fund and N. Auersperg for cell lines; Ed Harlow, E. Gurney, L. Gooding, R. Coffman, and G. Jay for monoclonal antibodies; David Pim for his expert technical assistance, and Penny Morgan for her help with the manuscript.

REFERENCES

1. Ahmad-Zadeh, C., Allet, B., Greenblatt, J., and Weil, R. (1976): Two forms of simian-virus-40-specific T-antigen in abortive and lytic infection. *Proc. Natl. Acad. Sci. USA*, 73:1097–1101.
2. Auersperg, J. (1964): Long-term cultivation of hypodiploid human tumor cells. *J. Natl. Cancer Inst.*, 32:135–163.
3. Carroll, R. B., Goldfine, S. M., and Melero, J. A. (1978): Antiserum to polyacrylamide gel-purified simian virus 40 T antigen. *Virology*, 87:194–198.
4. Carroll, R. B., and Smith, A. E. (1976): Monomer molecular weight of T antigen from simian virus 40-infected and transformed cells. *Proc. Natl. Acad. Sci. USA*, 73:2254–2258.
5. Cleveland, D. W., Fischer, S. G., Kirschner, M. W., and Laemmli, U. K. (1977): Peptide mapping by limited proteolysis in sodium dodecyl sulfate and analysis by gel electrophoresis. *J. Biol. Chem.*, 252:1102–1106.
6. Coffman, R. L., and Weissman, I. L. (1981): A monoclonal antibody that recognizes B cells and B cell precursors in mice. *J. Exp. Med.*, 153:269–279.

7. Crawford, L. V., Cole, C. N., Smith, A. E., Paucha, E., Tegtmeyer, P., Rundell, K., and Berg, P. (1978): Organization and expression of early genes of simian virus 40. *Proc. Natl. Acad. Sci. USA*, 75:117–121.

8. Crawford, L. V., Lane, D. P., Denhardt, D. T., Harlow, E. E., Nicklin, P. M., Osborn, K., and Pim, D. C. (1980): Characterization of the complex between SV40 large T antigen and the 53K host protein in transformed mouse cells. *Cold Spring Harbor Symp. Quant. Biol.*, 44:179–187.

9. Crawford, L., Leppard, K., Lane, D., and Harlow, E. (1982): Cellular proteins reactive with monoclonal antibodies directed against SV40 T-antigen. *J. Virology*, 42:612–620.

10. Crawford, L. V., Pim, D. C., Gurney, E. G., Goodfellow, P., and Taylor-Papadimitriou, J. (1981): Detection of a common feature in several human tumor cell lines: A 53,000-dalton protein. *Proc. Natl. Acad. Sci. USA*, 78:41–45.

11. Crawford, L. V., Pim, D. C., and Lane, D. P. (1979): An immunochemical investigation of SV40 T antigens. 2. Quantitation of antigens and antibody activities. *Virology*, 100:314–325.

12. DeLeo, A. B., Jay, G., Appella, E., Dubois, G. C., Law, L. W., and Old, L. J. (1979): Detection of a transformation-related antigen in chemically induced sarcomas and other transformed cells of the mouse. *Proc. Natl. Acad. Sci. USA*, 76:2420–2424.

13. Dippold, W. G., Jay, G., DeLeo, A. B., Khoury, G., and Old, L. J. (1981): p53 transformation-related protein: Detection by monoclonal antibodies in mouse and human cells. *Proc. Natl. Acad. Sci. USA*, 78:1695–1699.

14. Fiers, W., Contreras, R., Haegeman, G., Rogiers, R., Van de Voorde, A., Van Heuverswyn, H., Van Herreweghe, J., Volckaert, G., and Ysebaert, M. (1978): The complete nucleotide sequence of SV40 DNA. *Nature*, 272:113–120.

15. Gurney, E. G., Harrison, R. O., and Fenno, J. (1980): Monoclonal antibodies against simian virus 40 T antigens: Evidence for distinct subclasses of large T antigen and for similarities among nonviral T antigens. *J. Virol.*, 34:752–763.

16. Harlow, E., Crawford, L. V., Pim, D. C., and Williamson, N. M. (1981): Monoclonal antibodies specific for the SV40 tumor antigens. *J. Virol.*, 39:861–869.

17. Harlow, E., Pim, D. C., and Crawford, L. V. (1981): Complex of simian virus 40 large-T antigen and host 53,000 molecular weight protein in monkey cells. *J. Virol.*, 37:564–573.

18. Ito, Y., Brocklehurst, J. R., and Dulbecco, R. (1977): Virus-specific proteins in the plasma membrane of cells lytically infected or transformed by polyoma virus. *Proc. Natl. Acad. Sci. USA*, 74:4666–4670.

19. Ito, Y., Brocklehurst, J., Spurr, N., Griffiths, M., Hurst, J., and Fried, M. (1977): Polyoma virus wild-type and mutant T antigens. *INSERM Colloq.*, 69:145–152.

20. Lane, D. P., and Crawford, L. V. (1979): T antigen is bound to a host protein in SV40-transformed cells. *Nature*, 278:261–263.

21. Lane, D. P., and Hoeffler, W. K. (1980): SV40 large T shares an antigenic determinant with a cellular protein of molecular weight 68,000. *Nature*, 288:167–170.
22. Lane, D. P., and Robbins, A. K. (1978): An immunochemical investigation of SV40 T antigens. 1. Production, properties and specificity of a rabbit antibody to purified simian virus large T-antigen. *Virology*, 87:182–193.
23. Linzer, D. I. H., and Levine, A. J. (1979): Characterization of a 54K dalton cellular SV40 tumor antigen present in SV40-transformed cells and uninfected embryonal carcinoma cells. *Cell*, 17:43–52.
24. Marshall, C. J., Franks, L. M., and Carbonell, A. W. (1977): Markers of neoplastic transformation in epithelial cell lines derived from human carcinomas. *J. Natl. Cancer Inst.*, 58:1743–1747.
25. McCormick, F., and Harlow, E. (1980): Association of a murine 53,000 dalton phosphoprotein with simian virus 40 large-T antigen in transformed cells. *J. Virol.*, 34:213–224.
26. Melero, J. A., Stitt, D. T., Mangel, W. F., and Carroll, R. B. (1979): Identification of new polypeptide species (48–55K) immunoprecipitable by antiserum to purified large T antigen and present in SV40-infected and -transformed cells. *Virology*, 93:466–480.
27. O'Farrell, P. Z., Goodman, H. M., and O'Farrell, P. H. (1977): High resolution two-dimensional electrophoresis of basic as well as acidic proteins. *Cell*, 12:1133–1142.
28. Reddy, V. B., Thimmappaya, B., Dhar, R., Subramanian, K. N., Zain, B. S., Pan, J., Ghosh, P. K., Celma, M. L., and Weissman, S. M. (1978): The genome of simian virus 40. *Science*, 200:494–502.
29. Rotter, V., Witte, O. N., Coffman, R., and Baltimore, D. (1980): Abelson murine leukemia virus-induced tumors elicit antibodies against a host cell protein P50. *J. Virol.*, 36:547–555.
30. Rundell, K., Collins, J. K., Tegtmeyer, P., Ozer, H. L., Lai, C. J., and Nathans, D. (1977): Identification of simian virus 40 protein A. *J. Virol.*, 21:636–646.
31. Simmons, D. T., Martin, M. A., Mora, P. T., and Chang, C. (1980): Relationship among Tau antigens isolated from various lines of simian virus 40 transformed cells. *J. Virol.*, 34:650–657.
32. Tegtmeyer, P. (1975): Function of simian virus 40 gene A in transforming infection. *J. Virol.*, 15:613–618.

Advances in Viral Oncology, Volume 2, edited by
George Klein. Raven Press, New York © 1982.

The Complex Between p53 and SV40 T Antigen

D. P. Lane, J. Gannon, and G. Winchester

*Cancer Research Campaign, Eukaryotic Molecular Genetics Research Group,
Department of Biochemistry, Imperial College, London SW7, England*

VIRUS–HOST INTERACTIONS

Viruses are obligate parasites, as they are totally dependent on
the host cell for their propagation. They are of relatively simple
genetic constitution compared with the host cell, and yet they must
intimately interact with its machinery in order to divert the cells
metabolism to viral reproduction. The study of viruses and their
interaction with the host cell in both prokaryotic and eukaryotic
systems has been one of the most successful ways of determining
how cells work at the molecular level. The discovery of oncogenic
viruses with small genomes has long held out the hope of reaching
a molecular understanding of cancer, despite the lack of evidence
for a viral etiology in the vast majority of human neoplastic disease.
Most investigators feel that the oncogenic process must bear some
common molecular "fingerprint" whether caused by virus, chemical,
solid body, or radiation. The excitement that surrounds the study
of the p53 protein described in this chapter and several others in
this book stems from the hope that p53 might itself be just such a
fingerprint. The key questions to be asked about any molecule that
is associated with oncogenesis are, first, is it ubiquitous in tumors
and absent or different or depressed in all normal tissues, and second,

23

does the molecule have a causal role in the oncogenic process or is it a passive consequence? Neither of these questions has been fully answered yet for p53, but it has a set of intriguing properties that mesh with one's ideas of such a fingerprint molecule and encourage further investigation.

THE DISCOVERY OF p53

In 1979 a number of independent research groups working on transformation by SV40 of rodent cells in tissue culture reported that in addition to the two SV40 early region gene products already identified, small t and large T, these cells contained a third protein or set of proteins of approximately 53,000 molecular weight (4,11,20, 21,25,32,43). This third protein was detected because like large T and small t it was specifically immunoprecipitated by sera derived from SV40 tumor bearing hamsters and not by control sera. The nature of this protein and the reason for its presence in the immunoprecipitates became the subject of intense investigation, originally fired by the expectation that it was a third gene product encoded by the early region of the SV40 virus, since Ito et al. (17) had recently identified a third early region product from the related papovavirus, Polyoma.

We had already adopted an immunochemical approach to the study of the SV40 T antigens and, in particular, had prepared a rabbit antisera to large T antigen purified by immunoprecipitation and SDS gel electrophoresis from lytically infected cells (24). This antiserum had been characterized quite extensively and had demonstrated the presence on native T antigen molecules of a set of antigenic determinants resistnt to denaturation by SDS gel electrophoresis. The existence of these determinants allowed the establishment of radioimmunoassays using gel-purified T antigens and showed that large T and small t shared common antigenic determinants since they were both independently recognized by the anti-large T polypeptide serum. A number of other less prominent polypeptides immunoprecipitated from lytically infected cells were also found to be independently recognized by this serum. This gave us confidence that we could recognize large T related proteins. When this serum was used to precipitate ^{35}S met labeled extracts of SV40 transformed mouse cells (SVA31E7) a third band of molecular weight 53,000 was clearly specifically precipitated. However, when this 53,000 protein was eluted from the gel it could not be bound by the rabbit anti-T serum. The 53,000 protein was the first instance in which we detected such an anomaly, i.e., a protein that was specifically precipitated from native cell extracts but which could not be rebound by this anti-SDS denatured T antibody when eluted from the gel. This led us to consider the possibility that the p53 was precipitated from the cell extracts by the monospecific anti-T serum because it was physically complexed to the large T protein (21). Subsequent experiments fitted in very well with this hypothesis, since every anti-T serum we tested precipitated the p53 protein as well as large T. Furthermore, titrations of these different sera, in particular the monospecific anti-SDS T serum in the precipitation system, demonstrated that the ratio of large T to p53 brought down was constant over a wide range of serum dilutions. Most sera we tested behaved in a similar manner in that they could precipitate T and p53 from cell extracts but bound only large T when used in radioimmunoassay against the gel-purified proteins. One set of sera proved exceptional; they were able to bind to the gel-purified p53 as well as to the large T, although their titer against p53 was much lower than their anti-T titer. These sera had been produced by repeatedly immunizing adult Balb/c mice with syngeneic SV40-transformed cells (SVT2). Since the specific immunoprecipitation of p53 from SV40-transformed cells could be explained by the T-53 complex idea, and since p53 lacked any of the antigenic determinants detected by the anti-SDS T serum, we entertained the idea that the p53 protein might not be virus coded but rather a product of the host cell. We were fortunate to be able to test this critically, having found the mouse sera that could recognize p53 in the absence of any large T. These mouse sera were found to precipitate a specific 53,000 molecular weight protein from cells transformed by Polyoma virus which contained no SV40 virus information. On the basis of these results we suggested that p53 was a host cell protein that was bound to the SV40 large T in SV40-transformed mouse cells (5,8, 21,22).

A number of other groups simultaneously or very soon afterward came to similar conclusions about the host cell nature of the p53 protein, although the idea of its physically being complexed to large T was accepted more slowly. Of particular importance were two papers that came out within months of ours. The first, by Linzer and Levine (25), showed that p53 was present at high levels in undifferentiated embryonal carcinoma cells. These authors used the partial proteolysis method of Cleveland to establish that the p53 precipitated from SV40-transformed mouse cells was very closely related or identical to the p53 present in embryonal carcinoma cells, providing more convincing evidence than our study on the Polyoma transformants had for the host cell nature of the p53 protein. (Subsequent peptide mapping studies from our group confirmed the identity of p53s isolated from SV40- and Polyoma-transformed cells) (5). The second crucial study which generated enormous excitement in the field was published by De Leo et al. (9). They had hyperimmunized mice with a syngeneic methylcolanthrene induced tumor cell line, meth A, in part of a search for the elusive tumor specific transplantation antigens of chemically transformed cells. Remarkably, sera from these mice precipitated a p53 that was present in extracts of a wide variety of murine tumor cell lines, induced by chemicals, radiation, DNA or RNA tumor viruses, but was absent or undetectable in "normal" cell lines.

DEFINITION OF p53

Subsequent work published by a large number of groups and summarized in their respective chapters in this volume has led to an explosion in our knowledge about the p53 protein(s). It has also led to problems of definition, and it is not clear that every group is always working with the same polypeptide or family of polypeptides. Fortunately a reasonable set of criteria exists by which a prospective protein can be identified as p53-related (7,34). First, the protein should be capable of binding to SV40 large T antigen;

second, it should be reactive with the monoclonal antibodies PAb122 (14) and PAb421 (16); and finally, it should have a peptide map with a set of identifiable common peptides to a p53 standard or standards. While there are clear species differences between p53s in terms of molecular weight and peptide map, proteins that satisfy the three criteria have been found in human, monkey, hamster, rat, and mouse cells. Indeed, so far, they have been found in some cell lines derived from every mammalian species that has been looked at.

The question of definition is an important one and may explain some anomalous results obtained by different groups. None of these criteria stands by itself as a sufficient definition, as, for instance, monoclonal antibodies quite frequently react with other, otherwise unrelated, molecular species (1,6,10,23,39), and there may be other T binding proteins. The peptide mapping procedure is relatively laborious and dependent on the standard itself but is intrinsically the most definitive. The sort of problems that arise from the lack of definition of p53 are illustrated by the suggestion of surface expression of p53 dependent solely on a monoclonal antibody fluorescence assay. Here p53 was seen to be a surface and cytoplasmic protein, whereas most groups have identified it as a nuclear species (41). Similarly, the p53 species identified by Luka et al. (27) complexed to EBNA in EB-transformed human lymphocytes has not yet been rigorously identified as a member of the p53 family by the above criteria. Certain facts are, however, clearly established and these are listed in Table 1.

ASSAYS FOR THE T-p53 COMPLEX

Of particular interest to us has been the nature and purpose of the specific binding of T antigen to p53. The interaction is non-covalent. In rodent cells the binding is very tight and resistant to both reducing agents and high pH (34), whereas in human cells and monkey cells experiments have suggested that the association is weaker and more readily disrupted. To date, the region of T antigen responsible for 53K binding has not been identified and quantitative

TABLE 1. *A summary of the properties of p53*

---

1. p53 binds SV40 large T antigen and super T antigen *in vivo* (5,7,8, 12,15,20,21,22,31,34).
2. p53 binds SV40 large T antigen *in vitro* (33).
3. p53 from primates binds SV40 large T less tightly than p53 from rodents (12,14,15,22).
4. p53 is conserved in primary structure and antigenically among mammalian species (7,14,16,32,42,43).
5. p53 acts as an autoantigen in a variety of murine tumors induced by chemicals, RNA viruses, and DNA viruses (9,21,25,31,41).
6. p53 is phosphorylated (5,31).
7. p53 levels, detected by metabolic labeling, are higher in a variety of different transformed cells than in their normal untransformed counterparts (7,9,14,18,26,41).
8. p53 levels detected by metabolic labeling are increased by SV40 infection of permissive and nonpermissive cells (2,15,26).
9. p53 has a very short half-life in "normal" 3T3 cells, but a much longer half-life in SV40-transformed 3T3 cells, SV3T3 (38).
10. p53 translatable mRNA levels are similar in 3T3 and SV3T3 cells (38).
11. p53 synthesis follows ConA stimulation of lymphocytes (35,36).
12. p53 synthesis is detectable in normal thymus (18,41).
13. p53 synthesis is detectable in explants of early embryos (3,37).
14. p53 is undetectable in HeLa cells (7).

---

studies on the complex have been somewhat restricted by the need to metabolically label the proteins involved in order to detect it. We have developed radioimmunometric assays using monoclonal antibodies that are capable of measuring T antigen concentration, T-p53 complex, and free p53 in cell extracts. As an alternative approach we have combined immunoprecipitation and immunoblotting (44) procedures to examine the complex. Both techniques are quantitative, do not depend on metabolic labeling, and avoid washing procedures that might dissociate proteins that are weakly bound to each other. Part of the motivation for developing such methods is the belief that the T-p53 complex may represent only the tip of an iceberg, and that many other important protein-protein interactions between p53 and other molecules are waiting to be discovered. We have indeed previously put forward an evolutionary argument about the T-p53 interaction that led us to propose that p53 normally binds to a cellular structure (a T equivalent structure) and is displaced from this interaction by T antigen (22).

The principle of the radioimmunometric assays is illustrated in Fig. 1. PAb204 is an anti-T monoclonal antibody that binds to a denaturation resistant site located in the C terminal half of large T (23). The antibody binds to protein A only weakly, and in the conditions used for the assay it will not interact with protein A bearing *Staphylococcus aureus*. The antibody has a very high affinity for T and can be readily iodinated to high specific activity using a solid phase lactoperoxidase method. When a cell extract containing T antigen is incubated with ^{125}I PAb204 the T molecules are bound by the antibody. These complexes will still not bind to Staph A cells. However, if a second monoclonal antibody to T that binds to a discrete site and binds tightly to Staph A cells is introduced into the system, then the ^{125}I PAb204-T antigen complex will be bound through this antibody to the solid phase. The assay has proved

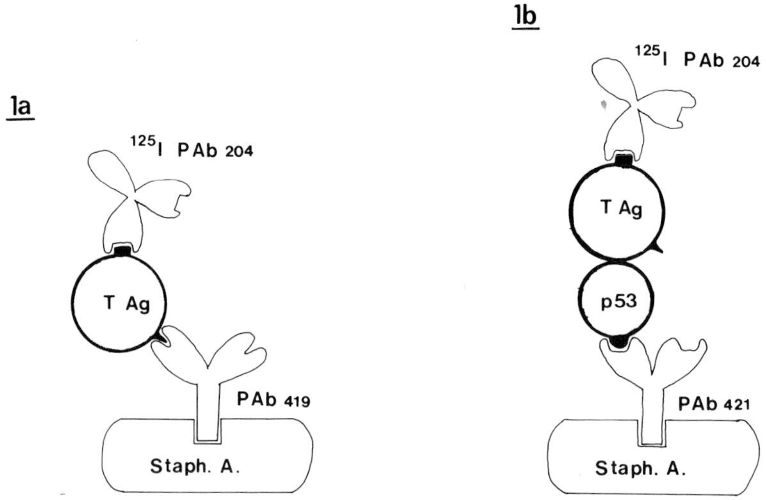

FIG. 1. Principle of radioimmunometric assays for SV40 large T and the T-p53 complex. **a:** Measurement of T—an anti-T monoclonal antibody, PAb204, that does not bind protein A is iodinated. The complex of this antibody with T antigen is precipitated by Staph A cells only in the presence of another unlabeled anti-T monoclonal, PAb419, that binds to a different site on T and binds Staph A cells. **b:** Measurement of T-p53 complex—iodinated PAb204 is bound by the complex, which can then be precipitated by Staph A cells in the presence of a Staph A binding anti-p53 monoclonal antibody, PAb421.

to be very versatile and accurate. It was initially set up as described
to measure T antigen; the sort of results obtained are illustrated in
Fig. 2. Here both the labeled antibody and the unlabeled antibody
are in excess. When cell extracts from mouse cells transformed by
SV40 are examined in this system the complex between T and 53K
can be readily measured using an unlabeled anti-53K monoclonal,
as illustrated in Fig. 1b. By measuring total T concentration as well
as the concentration of T which is bound to 53K in the same extract
it has been possible to rapidly compare different lines of SV40-
transformed cells for the amount of large T which is in the complex
versus the amount that is uncoupled to 53K. The assay does not

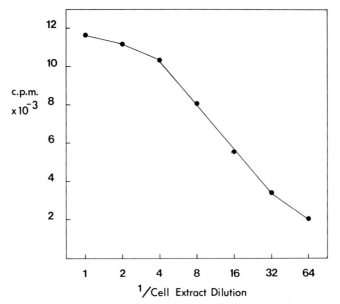

FIG. 2. Radioimmunometric assay of SV40 large T antigen. A cell extract was prepared by lysing 5×10^6 SV80 cells in 2 ml of buffer (1% NP40, 120 mM NaCl, 10 mM
Tris pH 8.0). 100 μl of a series of dilutions of this extract were mixed with 100 μl
(2×10^4 cpm) of ^{125}I PAb204. After 2 hr incubation 100 μl of PAb419 were added
and after a further 2 hr incubation 50 μl of a 10% suspension of Staph A cells was
added. Thirty minutes later the Staph A cells were harvested by centrifugation, washed
once in 1% NP40, 120 mM NaCl, 10 mM Tris pH 8.0 and counted in a gamma counter.
In the absence of cell extract containing T antigen about 500 cpm are bound non-
specifically in this system.

require any extensive washing procedure, unlike conventional immunoprecipitations, and it is not dependent on the incorporation of
metabolic label. Table 2 and Fig. 3 illustrate some of the results
we have obtained with this technique, which we are now applying
to the study of TsA mutant-transformed rodent cells. So far the

TABLE 2.

Cell line	% T bound to p53
SV3T3 Cl38	22%
SV3T3 ClM	35%
SV3T3 ClH	47%
SV3T3 Cl49	30%
*SV3T3 Cl20	72%

Ratios were determined at plateau values in which all antibodies were in excess
as illustrated in Fig. 3. The cell lines are as
described in Rigby et al. (40).

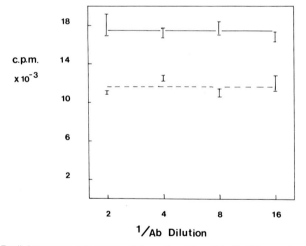

FIG. 3. Radioimmunometric assay of the ratio of free T to T-p53 complex in Clone
20, SV40 transformed mouse cells. In each tube a fixed volume (100 μl) of cell extract
prepared as in Fig. 1 from Clone 20 cells was incubated with 3 × 10⁴ cpm of PAb204.
Then varying dilutions of PAb419 (—) or PAb122 (-----) were added as indicated. The
graph shows the stability of the plateau value of T complex detected in antibody
excess.

results have been in broad agreement with those obtained by our-selves and others using sequential immunoprecipitation and sucrose gradient separations on metabolically labeled extracts (14,22,34). In general, around 50% of the T antigen is in the complexed form in mouse cells. Interestingly, in the Clone 20 cells, which make a super T antigen only (40), the proportion of T in the complex is notably greater. This result might be explained if the super T species has a higher affinity for p53 than the wild type protein. Indeed with a super T of a slightly different type the Mays have obtained evidence that p53 preferentially binds this species rather than wild type T (29,30). When extracts of human cells are examined using this assay technique a rather different picture emerges. Initially we were unable to detect any T antigen that could be precipitated with the anti-p53 monoclonals. However, if freshly prepared cell extracts were used rather than frozen and thawed ones, some complexes were detect-able. Careful titration of the anti-p53 antibody showed that the curve of precipitation by this species was very different from that seen in the rodent system. At saturation, however, all of the T molecules that were precipitated with anti-T monoclonals could also be pre-cipitated with anti-p53 monoclonals (Fig. 4). The need for such high relative concentrations of anti-p53 in the human system can be most simply explained either by a lower affinity of the antibody for human p53 than mouse p53, or by the presence of excess un-complexed p53 in the human system. Indeed, evidence for the ex-istence of free p53 in SV40-transformed human cells has been obtained by sequential immunoprecipitation studies (22). In mouse cells all available p53 seems to be complexed to T with free T molecules usually present as well. The state of the complex inside the cell is of course more difficult to measure as the concentrations of the two components will be much higher, and it is not clear that an equi-librium similar to that seen in these *in vitro* experiments would be reached. We hope in the future to use the assay to screen mutant cells, particularly SV40-transformed cells selected for reversion to normal growth, for alterations in the T-p53 complex in the hope of detecting revertants that have altered their p53 so that it no longer binds large T. In an earlier study (22) a few large T expressing

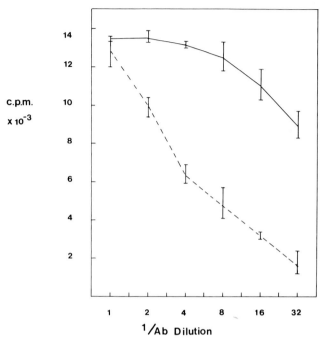

FIG. 4. Radioimmunometric assay of the ratio of free T to T-p53 complex in SV80; SV40-transformed human cells. The ratio of T to T-p53 was determined over a range of antibody concentrations, as in Fig. 3, with varying dilutions of PAb419 (—) and PAb122 (-----) added.

revertants were all found to still express p53 which was complexed to T, so that alterations in p53 are clearly not the only route to reversion, and cells can express high levels of p53 and yet still show "normal" growth control.

The radioimmunometric assay can also be used to screen sera for anti-p53 activity. Since in a variety of different murine tumor systems, anti-p53 antibodies are produced by tumor bearing animals, we embarked on a modest screen of human tumor patient serum samples using this and the immunoblot assays described below. So far, no serum out of the 20 tested has shown any titer at all.

Finally, we have used the radioimmunometric assay in competition measurements of free p53. In this system super T-p53 complexes from murine Clone 20 cells are labeled with PAb204 ^{125}I and their precipitation by anti-p53 monoclonal antibody (PAb421) (16) inhibited by cell extracts containing free p53. Although this test is rather complex in design, in practice it is simple to perform and shows good specificity. HeLa cell extracts, for instance, which contain no p53 reactive with PAb421 (7), do not inhibit binding at all in this system, whereas good inhibition curves are obtained with extracts of the p53 positive Namalva cell line.

As an alternative approach to the radioimmunometric assays for detection of T-p53 complexes we have also employed an immunoblotting technique (44). Here the sample to be analyzed is run in a standard SDS gel, and the separated proteins are transferred electrophoretically to nitrocellulose sheets. The location of the protein of interest is then determined by staining the sheet with antibody. Usually we use an enzyme-labeled second antibody or iodinated protein A as a detection system. The procedure works extremely well for T-antigen stained either with whole anti-T sera or with PAb204. It is disappointing that we have not obtained any positive signal with either of the P53 monoclonals available to us (PAb122 and PAb421); however, the system has been useful since immune precipitates of the T-p53 complex can be readily analyzed. In a practical test a cell extract would be precipitated with an anti-T antibody and a p53 antibody and the resultant precipitates analysed for T antigen using the immunoblot. The power of the technique is again that metabolic labeling is not required and the immunoprecipitate need not be washed because of the specificity of the detection system. Results obtained in these systems have been in broad agreement with earlier studies, but again it offers great promise when looking for weaker interactions. McCormick et al. (33) were able to show *in vitro* binding of p53 from F9 cells to purified T antigen. We have examined the possibility of using this *in vitro* binding to detect p53 binding proteins on immunoblots. In this system total cell extracts run in SDS gels are transferred to nitrocellulose, incubated with p53 containing cell extracts (i.e., from F9 cells), and the resulting filter stained with PAb421. As a control the filter is incubated in HeLa cell extracts. Using this system we have obtained preliminary results which indicate that the major p53 binding protein apart from large T (where present) is p53 itself! However, further work is needed to validate this finding.

DISCUSSION

The p53 protein is as yet poorly understood. Its tight binding to SV40 T antigen suggested that it might play a role in transformation by this virus, and the discovery that it was present in elevated levels in tumors induced by other agents hinted that it might play a more general role. There is not yet sufficient data to evaluate whether p53 plays any causal role in the oncogenic process or merely reflects the altered metabolism of the transformed cell. The important experiments of Oren et al. (38) showed that p53 in 3T3 cells has an extremely short half-life, whereas in SV40-transformed 3T3 cells the half-life is greatly increased. In this system at least, then, p53 concentration in a cell population is controlled by posttranslational mechanisms rather than at the transcriptional level. It is clearly of key importance to determine whether p53 concentration in other tumor cell systems is also regulated in this way. The very short half-life of the protein suggests that it may play a specific regulatory role in the cell. Since SV40 large T is known to be involved in the initiation of both viral and cellular DNA synthesis, it is reasonable to speculate that p53 may have a normal role to play in cell DNA synthesis. It is clear that more direct experiments are needed to get at the function of p53; purifying the protein and cloning the p53 gene will provide the necessary tools. The key question of whether p53 is a passive indicator or an active cause of cellular transformation will then be answerable. Crawford et al. (7) have shown increased synthesis and/or accumulation of p53 to be a common feature of cell lines recently derived from human neoplasms, and this suggests that measurement of p53 and perhaps anti-p53 antibody may have clinical significance. The assays described here represent one approach toward these problems, but they have not as yet provided any novel insights. We strongly suspect, however, that the large T p53 interaction represents an extreme case of protein-protein interaction between an oncogenic virus and the host cell, and we hope that the sensitive methods we are developing will reveal many more such interactions.

ACKNOWLEDGMENTS

We thank Ed Harlow and Tucker Gurney for gifts of monoclonal antibodies without which these experiments could not have been done. We also thank David Pim, Alan Robbins, and Warren Hoeffler for valuable technical assistance in the early experiments discussed here. Finally we thank all our colleagues at the I.C.R.F., Cold Spring Harbor, and Imperial College for many helpful discussions and encouragement. Special thanks are due to Lionel Crawford and Ed Harlow. This research is supported by a grant from the Cancer Research Campaign.

REFERENCES

1. Blose, S. H., Matsumura, F., and Lin, J. J. C. (1981): The structure of vimentin-10 nm filaments probed with a monoclonal antibody that recognises a common antigenic determinant on vimentin and tropomyosin. *Cold Spring Harbor Symp. Quant. Biol.*, 49: (*in press*).
2. Carroll, R. B., Muello, K., and Melero, J. A. (1980): Coordinate expression of the 48K host nuclear phosphoprotein and SV40 T Ag upon primary infection of mouse cells. *Virology*, 102:447–452.
3. Chandrasekaran, K., McFarland, V. W., Simmons, D. T., Dziadek, M., Gurney, E. G., and Mora, P. T. (1981): Quantitation and characterisation of a species specific and embryo age dependent 55K M.W. phosphoprotein which is also present in cells transformed by SV40. *Proc. Natl. Acad.Sci. USA*, 78:6953–6957.
4. Chang, C., Simmons, D. T., Martin, M. A., and Mora, P. T. (1979): Identification and partial characterisation of new antigens from simian virus 40-transformed mouse cells. *J. Virol.*, 31:463–471.
5. Crawford, L. V., Lane, D. P., Danhardt, D. T., Harlow, E. E., Nicklin, P. M., Osborn, K., and Pim, D. C. (1980): Characterisation of the complex between SV40 large T antigen and the 53K host protein in transformed mouse cells. *Cold Spring Harbor Symp. Quant. Biol.*, 44:179–187.
6. Crawford, L., Leppard, K., Lane, D., and Harlow, E. (1982): Cellular proteins reactive with monoclonal antibodies directed against SV40 T-antigen. *J. Virol.*, 42:612–620.
7. Crawford, L. V., Pim, D. C., Gurney, E. G., Goodfellow, P., and Taylor-Papadimitriou, J. (1981): Detection of a common feature in several human

tumor cell lines: a 53,000 dalton protein. *Proc. Natl. Acad. Sci. USA*, 78:41–45.

8. Crawford, L. V., Pim, D. C., and Lane, D. P. (1980): An immunochemical investigation of SV40 T-antigens 2. Quantitation of antigens and antibody activities. *Virology*, 100:314–325.
9. DeLeo, A. B., Jay, G., Appella, E., Dubois, G. C., Law, L. W., and Old, L. J. (1979): Detection of a transformation related antigen in chemically induced sarcomas and other transformed cells of the mouse. *Proc. Natl. Acad. Sci. USA*, 76:2420–2424.
10. Dulbecco, R., Unger, M., Bologna, M., Battifora, H., Syka, P., and Okada, S. (1981): Cross reactivity between Thy-1 and a component of intermediate filaments demonstrated using a monoclonal antibody. *Nature*, 292:772–774.
11. Edwards, C. A. F., Khoury, G., and Martin, R. G. (1979): Phosphorylation of T-antigen and control of T antigen expression in cells transformed by wild-type and tsA mutants of simian virus 40. *J. Virol.*, 29:753–762.
12. Fanning, E., Nowak, B., and Burger, C. (1981): Detection and characterisation of multiple forms of simian virus 40 large T antigen. *J. Virol.*, 37:92–102.
13. Greenspan, D. S., and Carroll, R. B. (1981): Complex of simian virus 40 large T antigen and 48,000 dalton host tumor antigen. *Proc. Natl. Acad. Sci. USA*, 78:105–109.
14. Gurney, E. G., Harrison, R. O., and Fenno, J. (1980): Monoclonal antibodies against simian virus 40 T antigens: evidence for distinct subclasses of large T antigen and for similarities among nonviral T antigens. *J. Virol.*, 34:752–763.
15. Harlow, E., Pim, D. C., and Crawford, L. V. (1981): Complex of simian virus 40 large T antigen and host 53,000 molecular weight protein in monkey cells. *J. Virol.*, 37:564–573.
16. Harlow, E., Crawford, L. V., Pim, D. C., and Williamson, N. M. (1981): Monoclonal antibodies specific for simian virus 40 tumour antigens. *J. Virol.*, 39:861–869.
17. Ito, Y., Brocklehurst, J. R., and Dulbecco, R. (1977): Virus specific proteins in the plasma membrane of cells lytically infected or transformed by polyoma virus. *Proc. Natl. Acad. Sci. USA*, 74:1259.
18. Jay, G., DeLeo, A. B., Appella, E., Dubois, G. C., Law, L. W., Khoury, G., and Old, L. J. (1979): A common protein in murine sarcomas and leukemias. *Cold Spring Harbor Symp. Quant. Biol.*, 44:659–664.
19. Jay, G., Khoury, G., DeLeo, A. B., Dippold, W. G., and Old, L. J. (1981): p53 transformation-related protein: detection of an associated phosphotransferase activity. *Proc. Natl. Acad. Sci. USA*, 78:2932–2936.
20. Kress, M., May, E., Cassingena, R., and May, P. (1979): Simian virus 40 transformed cells express new species of proteins precipitable by anti simian virus 40 tumor serum. *J. Virol.*, 31:472–483.
21. Lane, D. P., and Crawford, L. V. (1979): T antigen is bound to a host protein in SV40-transformed cells. *Nature*, 278:261–263.

22. Lane, D. P., and Crawford, L. V. (1980): The complex between simian virus 40 T antigen and a specific host protein. *Proc. R. Soc. Lond. (Biol.)*, 210:451–453.

23. Lane, D. P., and Hoeffler, W. K. (1980): SV40 large T shares an antigenic determinant with a cellular protein of molecular weight 68,000. *Nature*, 288:167–170.

24. Lane, D. P., and Robbins, A. K. (1978): An immunochemical investigation of SV40 T-antigens. 1. Production, properties and specificity of a rabbit antibody to purified simian virus 40 large T antigen. *Virology*, 87:182–193.

25. Linzer, D. I. H., and Levine, A. J. (1979): Characterisation of a 54K dalton cellular SV40 tumor antigen present in SV40-transformed cells and uninfected embryonal carcinoma cells. *Cell*, 17:43–52.

26. Linzer, D. I. H., Maltzman, W., and Levine, A. J. (1979): The SV40 A gene product is required for the production of a 54,000 M.W. cellular tumor antigen. *Virology*, 98:308–318.

27. Luka, J., Jornvall, H., and Klein, G. (1980): Purification and biochemical characterisation of the Epstein-Barr virus-determined nuclear antigen and an associated protein with a 53,000 dalton subunit. *J. Virol.*, 35:592–602.

28. Maltzman, W., Oren, M., and Levine, A. J. (1981): The structural relationships between 54,000 molecular weight cellular tumor antigens detected in viral and nonviral transformed cells. *Virology*, 112:145–156.

29. May, E., Jeltsch, J. M., and Gannon, F. (1981): Characterisation of a gene encoding a 115K super T antigen expressed by a SV40 transformed rat cell line. *Nucleic Acids Res.*, 9:4111–4128.

30. May, E., Kress, M., Daya-Grosjean, L., Monier, R., and May, P. (1981): Mapping of the viral mRNA encoding a super T antigen of 115,000 daltons expressed in SV40-transformed rat cell lines. *J. Virol.*, 37:24–35.

31. May, P., Kress, M., Lange, M., and May, E. (1980): New genetic information expressed in SV40 transformed cells: Characterisation of the 55K proteins and evidence for unusual SV40 mRNAs. *Cold Spring Harbor Symp. Quant. Biol.*, 44:189–200.

32. Melero, J. A., Stitt, D. T., Mangel, W. F., and Carroll, R. B. (1979): Identification of new polypeptide species (48–55K) immunoprecipitable by antiserum to purified large T antigen and present in SV40 infected and transformed cells. *Virology*, 93:466–480.

33. McCormick, F., Clark, R., Harlow, E., and Tjian, R. (1981): SV40 T antigen binds specifically to a cellular 53K protein *in vitro*. *Nature*, 292:63–65.

34. McCormick, F., and Harlow, E. (1980): Association of a murine 53,000 dalton phosphoprotein with simian virus 40 large-T antigen in transformed cells. *J. Virol.*, 34:213–224.

35. Milner, J., and McCormick, F. (1980): Lymphocyte stimulation: Concanavalin A induces the expression of a 53K protein. *Cell Biol. Int. Rep.*, 4:663–667.

36. Milner, J., and Milner, S. (1981): SV40 53K antigen: a possible role for 53K in normal cells. *Virology*, 112:785–788.

37. Mora, P. T., Chandrasekaran, K., and McFarland, V. W. (1980): An embryo protein induced by SV40 virus transformation of mouse cells. *Nature*, 288:722–724.
38. Oren, M., Maltzman, W., and Levine, A. J. (1981): Post-translational regulation of the 54K cellular tumor antigen in normal and transformed cells. *Mol. Cell. Biochem.*, 1:101–110.
39. Pillemer, E., and Weissman, I. L. (1981): A monoclonal antibody that detects a V_k-TEPC15 idiotypic determinant cross-reactive with a Thy-1 determinant. *J. Exp. Med.*, 153:1068–1079.
40. Rigby, P. W. J., Chia, W., Clayton, C. E., and Lovett, M. (1980): The structure and expression of the integrated viral DNA in mouse cells transformed by simian virus 40. *Proc. R. Soc. Lond. (Biol.)*, 210:437–450.
41. Rotter, V., Boss, M. A., and Baltimore, D. (1981): Increased concentration of an apparently identical cellular protein in cells transformed by either Abelson murine leukemia virus or other transforming agents. *J. Virol.*, 38:336–346.
42. Simmons, D. T., Martin, M. A., Mora, P. T., and Chang, C. (1980): Relationship among Tau antigens isolated from various lines of simian virus 40 transformed cells. *J. Virol.*, 34:650–657.
43. Smith, A. E., Smith, R., and Paucha, E. (1979): Characterisation of different tumor antigens present in cells transformed by simian virus 40. *Cell*, 18:335–346.
44. Towbin, H., Staehelin, T., and Gordon, J. (1979): Electrophoretic transfer of proteins from polyacrylamide gels to nitrocellulose sheets: Procedure and some applications. *Proc. Natl. Acad. Sci. USA*, 76:4350–4354.

Advances in Viral Oncology, Volume 2, edited by
George Klein. Raven Press, New York © 1982.

Monoclonal Antibody Analysis of p53

Elizabeth G. Gurney

Department of Biology, University of Utah, Salt Lake City, Utah 84112

A phosphoprotein with monomer molecular weight of about 53,000 daltons (p53) has caught the attention of biologists interested in the malignant transformation. p53 was detected initially by virtue of its tight association with the large T antigen of simian virus 40 (SV40) in SV40-transformed cells but was shown to be a cellular rather than a viral tumor antigen and to be present at comparable levels in mammalian cells transformed by several agents (3,5,17,18,20,28). In the presumably untransformed cell line 3T3, p53 content is about 20-fold lower than in transformed cells, but rises to the transformed level after SV40 infection (21). Further study of this transformation-associated protein seems warranted and is underway in many laboratories. Different groups have called this protein various names such as nonviral tumor antigen, tau antigen, and 53K protein, but I will refer to it as p53 in this chapter.

Detection and purification of p53 currently depend on immunological methods. No biological functions or biochemical activities for p53 have yet been proven, although Jay et al. (15) recently reported that immune complexes containing p53 have protein kinase activity. Furthermore, p53 is a minor protein representing at most 1 part in 10,000 of cellular proteins. Therefore, p53 is identified by its presence in complexes with large T antigen in SV40-transformed cells or by its monomer molecular weight of 48,000 to 56,000 daltons after precipitation with particular antibody preparations. Sera from mice or hamsters immunized with SV40-transformed cells (18), from mice immunized with methylcholanthrene-induced tumor cells (5), or from rabbits immunized with electro-phoretically purified mouse p53 (22) have been used to study p53 proteins. However, monoclonal antibodies specific for p53 are now available (8,13,14,26) and promise to be more specific, more con-sistent, and of higher titer than any of the polyclonal sera. I will describe here an initial analysis of p53 using monoclonal antibody PAb122 that was isolated in my laboratory.

MONOCLONAL ANTIBODY PAb122

Robert Harrison, James Fenno, Susan Tamowski, and I have made clones of antibody secreting cells with the goal of collecting a set of monoclonal antibodies specific for the SV40 tumor antigens. We have used the procedure of Köhler and Milstein (16) to produce antibody-secreting hybrid cells by fusion of NS1 BALB/c myeloma cells with spleen cells from BALB/c mice immunized with live SV40-transformed cells of BALB/c origin. The parent NS1 (nonse-cretory) produces no detectable antibody despite its myeloma origin. Hybrid clones made by fusing NS1 with random spleen lymphocytes from a recently immunized mouse have the double attributes of indefinite and rapid growth in culture, acquired from the NS1, and secretion of a specific immunoglobulin, acquired from the particular fused spleen cell. The fusion process itself is not discriminating, and therefore many different fusion hybrids are formed. The suc-cessful isolation of a desired antibody-producing clone depends on the design of a screening or selection strategy to pick out one clone among the hundreds or thousands of possible hybrids. In our case, hybrid cells were screened for release of antibody able to bind to methanol-fixed SV40-transformed human cells (SV80) in an en-zyme-linked immunosorbent assay (ELISA) (9,13). Using the ELISA, we could detect hybrid cells secreting antibodies specific for tumor antigens when the antibody producers were present only as less than one-one hundredth of the population in a mixed "mass" culture. Mass cultures that gave positive results in the ELISA were cloned in soft agar and retested. A photograph of a typical screening assay is shown in Fig. 1. Positive clones were characterized using three

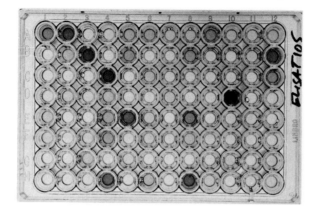

FIG. 1. Screening by ELISA. SV80 cells (6 × 10⁴ cells/well) were seeded in 96 microtiter wells and grown for one day. For fixation, the cells were rinsed once with PBS + 1% calf serum and once with methanol, soaked 5 min in fresh methanol, blown dry with air, and stored at −20° C. Before use, the wells were filled with distilled water at 22° C. The water was removed after 5 min and 50 μl medium samples were put into the wells. Wells A1 and A2 received medium from PAb100 (formerly known as clone 7) (13) cells as positive control. Wells A3 and A4 received medium from NS1 cells as negative control. The remaining wells received medium from the mass cultures resulting from two fusions. The medium was aspirated out of the wells after 60 min at 22° C, and the wells were rinsed three times with PBS + 0.05% Tween 20. Alkaline phosphatase-conjugated goat anti-mouse immunoglobulin G antibody (9), 50 μl of a 10-fold diluted solution per well, was added. After 24 hr at 22° C, the wells were rinsed three times with PBS + 0.05% Tween 20 before addition of 200 μl per well of alkaline phosphatase substrate (30). After 60 min at 22° C, 25 μl of 4 N NaOH were added to each well. The transilluminated plate was photographed through a Wratten 36 filter with Panatomic X (Kodak) film.

further tests, in order of increasing specificity: (a) immunofluorescence on fixed cells, both transformed and untransformed; (b) immunoprecipitation and electrophoretic analysis of radiolabeled proteins extracted from cells, both transformed and untransformed; and (c) immunoprecipitation of electrophoretically purified radiolabeled SV40 large T antigen and human or mouse p53. As shown in Table 1, we have obtained 15 clones of known specificity. Ten clones secrete antibodies that bind SV40 large T antigens, the specificity expected with our immunization and screening procedures. In addition to clones of the expected specificity, we found 4 clones that secrete antibodies that stain cytoplasmic structural components known as 10 nm filaments in immunofluorescence assays of a wide variety

TABLE 1. *Monoclonal antibody secreting clones produced*

No. clones	Specificity	Designation
10	Anti-SV40 T antigen	PAb100-109
1	Anti-p53	PAb122
4	Anti-10 nm filaments	666,773,817,914

of cells, whether transformed or not. Finally, we found a clone, PAb122, that secretes antibody recognizing p53 from 5 species of mammalian cells. PAb122 will be the focus of this article.

Isolation

The isolation and initial characterization of PAb122 have been described briefly (13) but will be described more fully here. BALB/c mice were injected subcutaneously at both 7 weeks of age and 13 weeks of age with 10^6 3T3/SV40 clone 4 (24) BALB/c cells. The mice did not develop tumors but did develop immunity to SV40 T antigens, which persisted for at least 6 months as shown by ELISA or immunofluorescence assay using mouse serum. Four months after the second injection, one mouse was given a subcutaneous injection of 3 to 4 $\times$ 10^7 3T3/SV40 clone 4 cells. Four days later the mouse was killed, the spleen excised, and 10^8 spleen cells were fused with 10^7 NS1 myeloma cells using PEG 1000 (Baker) as described by Galfrè et al. (11). Hybrid cells were selected in HAT medium in 48 mass cultures as described by Galfrè et al. (20). Cells in one mass culture were strongly positive in the ELISA 17 days after the fusion and were seeded in soft agar. Clones were transferred to liquid medium after 10 to 11 days growth in agar. More than half (163/288) of the clones tested by ELISA after several days' growth were strongly positive. Of the positive clones, 24 were saved but only 2 were characterized. These 2 clones gave identical results in all subsequent assays and both were called clone 122, and are now known as PAb122.

Growth

PAb122 cells are somewhat larger (perhaps double in volume) and more difficult to grow than our other hybrid cells. The cells grow with a doubling time of about 1 day from a density of 10^4 cells/ml to a density of about 5×10^5 cells/ml in Dulbecco's modification of Eagles' medium containing either 20% fetal calf serum or 10% calf serum plus 10% horse serum. The cells grow best as unstirred suspensions in bacterial Petri dishes. We found that, unlike NS1 cells or other hybrid cells, PAb122 cells did not grow well in glass or tissue culture-treated plastic containers and that many PAb122 cells attached to the surface of such containers. Relative antibody titers of medium samples were determined using the ELISA. As with other hybrid cells, the highest antibody titers seemed to be obtained by harvesting the medium a few days after the cells reached a high density and began to die. Sodium azide (1 to 4 mM final concentration) was added to medium samples after removal of cells and cellular debris by centrifugation (2,000 $\times$ g, 20° C, 2 min). Antibody titers were stable at 2 to 4° C for up to several months or at $-20°$ C for longer periods. Concentrated medium samples were prepared from 5 to 10 ml samples using Minicon B125 (Amicon) disposable concentrators or on a larger scale using ammonium sulfate at 50% saturation for precipitation.

Hybridoma serum was prepared from mice bearing subcutaneous PAb122 tumors. Unfortunately, hybridoma serum was not as useful as culture medium for our purposes, so I cannot recommend it. However, I can report that clone PAb122 did form hybridomas in two of the five BALB/c mice, each injected subcutaneously with 8×10^6 cells. Both tumors grew slowly, reaching 5 to 10 cm^3 by 10 weeks after injection. Tumor cells were transferred several times successively and appeared to become more tumorigenic. For example, all of the five BALB/c mice injected with 2×10^6 cells from one of the second passage tumors developed large tumors at the site of injection within 3 weeks. Cells from a subcutaneous tumor were also injected into the peritoneum of Pristane- (Aldrich-) treated BALB/c mice. Solid tumors developed slowly in the peritoneum of four out of the five injected mice. Ascitic fluid from these mice contained PAb122 antibody but at a lower titer than in the serum of animals with subcutaneous tumors. In the ELISA, the relative titer of PAb122 antibodies in serum from mice with sub–cutaneous tumors was approximately 100 times the antibody titer found with medium samples. In immunofluorescence assays, PAb122 medium could be diluted 20-fold without loss of typical nuclear fluorescence, whereas PAb122 serum could be diluted 2,000 to 5,000-fold. However, as shown in Fig. 2, the background cyto-plasmic fluorescence was higher for serum samples than for medium samples with equivalent nuclear fluorescence. Thus, the monoclonal antibody gave cleaner results in the absence of additional mouse antibodies.

Characterization

The specificity of PAb122 antibody for the cellular protein p53 was discovered using the radioimmunoassay developed by Lane and Robbins (19). Electrophoretically purified ^{35}S-labeled mouse p53 and SV40 large T antigen prepared by Lionel Crawford were in-cubated with antibodies. Immune complexes were precipitated with formalin-fixed *Staphylococcus aureus* Cowan I and counted by liq-uid scintillation methods. As shown in Table 2, PAb122 antibody bound gel-purified denatured mouse p53. In radioimmunoassays and in other immunoprecipitations, the PAb122 antibody was readily bound by fixed *Staphylococcus* or by *Staphylococcus* protein A bound to Sepharose (Pharmacia). Ochterlony double diffusion anal-ysis with class- and subclass-specific antibodies (kindly performed by Cliff Stocks and Seth Pincus) indicated that PAb122 antibodies are IgG$_{2b}$ molecules.

ANALYSIS OF p53

Cellular Distribution

PAb122 antibody recognizes a determinant shared by the p53 proteins of five mammalian species. Large T antigen and 51 to 56K

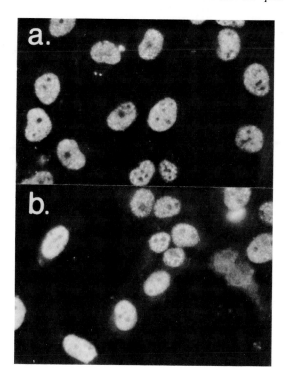

FIG. 2. Immunofluorescent comparison of PAb122 medium and serum. Subconfluent SV80 cells growing on glass coverslips were fixed with acetone-ethanol (2:1) for 20 min at 4° C (1) and assayed by indirect immunofluorescence (12). The first antibody used was **(a)** PAb122 medium (undiluted) or **(b)** PAb122 serum diluted 50-fold in PBS. Similar results were obtained with serum diluted 100 to 500-fold. Both coverslips were subsequently exposed to fluoresceinated goat anti-mouse immunoglobulin G antibody (Antibodies, Inc., 1/150 dilution in PBS) and photographed at ASA 1000 (Kodak Tri-X Pan film and Acufine developer) through a Zeiss microscope equipped for fluorescein epifluorescence.

p53 proteins were precipitated by PAb122 antibody from extracts of SV40-transformed human (13, Fig. 3a), rat (13, Fig. 3c), mouse (13), monkey (13, Figs. 3e and 3f), and hamster (SV40-transformed hamster embryo fibroblasts derived by Frank O'Neill and H65/90B obtained from Lionel Crawford, *data not shown*) cells. We found that human and mouse p53 proteins precipitated with PAb122 yielded peptides of similar sizes after partial digestion with *S. aureus* V8 protease (*data not shown*). Simmons (27) has recently shown by

TABLE 2. *Radioimmunoassay*

Antibody source	^{35}S-protein bound (cpm)	
	SV40 large T antigen[a]	Mouse p53[a]
Normal mouse serum	64	68
Serum from mouse used as spleen donor for PAb122	196 (27%)	198 (25%)
Serum from mouse bearing SVT2 tumor	340 (46%)	575 (74%)
PAb122 medium	95	438 (56%)
NS1 medium	92	93
Total cpm/sample	738	777

[a]Gifts from Lionel Crawford.

two-dimensional tryptic peptide mapping that the p53 proteins of monkey, human, mouse, and rat cells are not identical but have extensive regions of homology. We conclude that PAb122 antibody is specific for a denaturation-resistant determinant in a conserved region of p53.

Using PAb122 antibody, p53 proteins have been found in many but not all transformed or tumor cells analyzed. Varda Rotter and David Baltimore (*personal communication*) have precipitated p53 from Abelson murine leukemia virus-transformed mouse cells with PAb122 antibody. As shown in Fig. 4, PAb122 antibody precipitated p53 proteins from three spontaneously transformed cells derived from three different mouse strains—L929 (C3H), 3T6 (Swiss), and BALB/3T12 (BALB/c). Crawford et al. (4) found that PAb122 antibody precipitated p53 proteins from 12 of the 13 human tumor cell lines examined but from none of the 3 human normal cell strains tested. No p53 was detectable in HeLa cells by immunoprecipitation with SV40 tumor serum (13) or with PAb122 antibody (4,13, Fig. 3b) even after infection with adenovirus-SV40 hybrid viruses (6). However, another human cervical carcinoma cell line did have p53 (4).

The p53 protein is not restricted to transformed cells. Low levels have been detected in the BALB/3T3 cell line (13,21) and in early passage mouse embryo primary cultures (23,25). Larger amounts

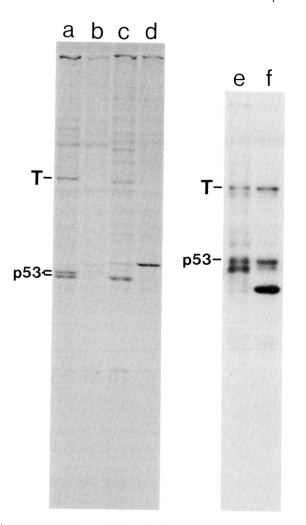

FIG. 3. Immunoprecipitation with PAb122 of extracts from human, rat, and monkey cells. Cellular proteins were labeled for 2 hr with ^{35}S-methionine in methionine-free medium, extracted with 1% Nonidet P40, 150 mM NaCl, 20 mM Tris pH 8.0, and immunoprecipitated with PAb122 medium as described previously (13). Precipitated proteins were eluted with sodium dodecyl sulfate and separated electrophoretically on a 7.5 to 15% acrylamide gradient slab gel. Cells used were **(a)** SV80, **(b)** HeLa, **(c)** 1_1 (SV40-transformed rat line derived by Michele Fluck), and **(d)** F111, the untransformed parent of 1_1 and monkey TC-7 cells infected with SV40 (m.o.i. about 35), and labeled **(e)** 15 to 17 hr postinfection (early) or **(f)** 39 to 41 hr postinfection (late).

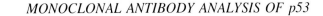

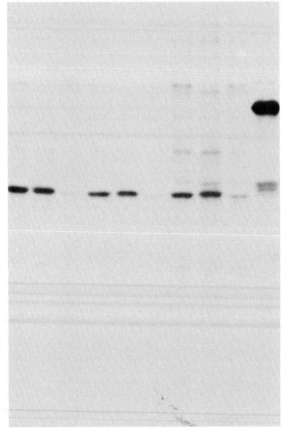

FIG. 4. Immunoprecipitation of extracts from spontaneously transformed mouse cells. Cellular proteins were labeled and extracted as in Fig. 3. Extracts were exposed to medium from hybrid cell clones or to SV40 tumor serum, and bound proteins were precipitated and analyzed as in Fig. 3. PAb101 (formerly known as clone 412) (13) antibody is specific for SV40 large T antigen. L929 cell extract precipitated with **(a)** tumor serum, **(b)** PAb122 medium, or **(c)** PAb101 medium; 3T6 cell extract precipitated with **(d)** tumor serum, **(e)** PAb122 medium, or **(f)** PAb101 medium; BALB/3T12 cell extract precipitated with **(g)** tumor serum, **(h)** PAb122 medium, or **(i)** PAb101 medium; and **(j)** SV80 cell extract precipitated with PAb101 medium.

of p53, comparable to those in transformed cells, have been found in primary cultures established from midgestation mouse, hamster, and rat embryos (2).

Cellular Location

By indirect immunofluorescence of fixed cells, we have found p53 to be a nuclear antigen. With SV40-transformed cells, the pattern of immunofluorescence was the same with PAb122 antibody, SV40 tumor serum, and monoclonal antibodies specific for SV40 large T antigen; the nucleoplasm of cells was fluorescent whereas nucleoli and metaphase chromosomes were dark. Typical staining of SV40-transformed human cells with PAb122 antibody is shown in Fig. 2. Similar results have been obtained with rabbit antiserum against electrophoretically purified mouse p53 (22) and with another monoclonal antibody specific for p53 (8). We found the same pattern of immunofluorescence with PAb122 on BALB/3T12 cells and on BALB/3T3 cells (Fig. 5). However, in the case of BALB/3T3, only 15 to 30% of the cells in a recently cloned population had fluorescent nuclei rather than every cell as seen with other cell lines. The reason for partial fluorescence in BALB/3T3 cells is not clear. We first surmised that p53 became prominent in certain phases of the cell

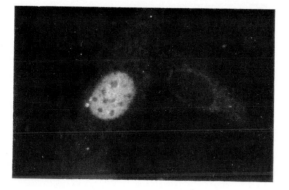

FIG. 5.   Immunofluorescence of PAb122 on BALB/3T3 cells. Sparse BALB/3T3 cells were fixed and assayed as in Fig. 2a.

cycle, but we have not been able to confirm this hypothesis using synchronized BALB/3T3 cultures. Both sparse, rapidly dividing BALB/3T3 and dense, "contact-inhibited" cultures showed the partial fluorescence.

Some p53 may be on the surface of SV40-transformed cells in addition to the nuclear p53. SV40 large T antigen is predominantly nuclear but is also present on the surface of transformed cells (7,29). Preliminary results obtained by Myriam Santos and Janet Butel (*personal communication*) indicate that p53 and SV40 large T antigen are tightly associated on the surface of SV40-transformed mouse cells. They were able to iodinate both proteins using a lactoperoxidase-catalyzed surface iodination procedure and to precipitate both proteins by either rabbit antiserum against purified large T antigen or PAb122 antibody.

Complexes with T Antigen

The tight association of p53 with large T antigen in SV40-transformed cells can be used to identify p53 and to provide clues to its function. As an example of this strategy, we used PAb122 antibody to determine the fraction of large T antigen and p53 present in T-p53 complexes. All antigens recognized by either anti-T or anti-p53 were removed by sequential immunoprecipitation of one sample of cell extract with four exposures to fresh antibody of one type. Then the remaining soluble antigens were exposed to the other type of antibody. Figure 6 shows the results obtained in reciprocal sequential precipitations of extract from SV80 cells labeled for 2 hr with ^{32}P-labeled inorganic phosphate using SV40 tumor serum (anti-T antibodies) and PAb122 medium (anti-p53 antibody). About 80% of the ^{32}P-labeled p53 was found in T-p53 complexes (Fig. 6a compared to Fig. 6d) whereas only about 20% of the ^{32}P-labeled large T antigen was in T-p53 complexes (Fig. 6e compared to Fig. 6h). Similar results were obtained with extracts of SV80 cells labeled for 2 hr with ^{35}S-methionine (10). Experiments are now in progress using longer labeling periods. Fanning et al. (10) found that complexes of large T antigen with p53 in extracts from mouse cells were more

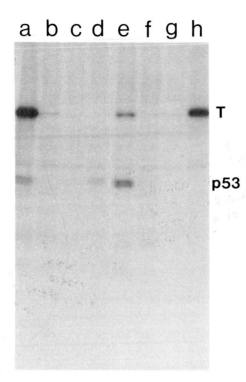

FIG. 6. Sequential immunoprecipitation of a ^{32}P-labeled SV80 cell extract. An extract of SV80 cells that had been labeled for 140 min with 200 μCi ^{32}PO$_4$ $^=$ in 1 ml phosphate-free medium was exposed to mouse SV40 tumor serum or to PAb122 medium that had been concentrated 10-fold using a Minicon B125 (Amicon) concentrator, and bound proteins were precipitated with *Staphylococcus*. Unbound proteins were exposed to another antibody sample in the same manner. Precipitated proteins were eluted with sodium dodecyl sulfate and electrophoretically separated on a 10% acrylamide slab gel. First **(a)**, second **(b)**, and fourth **(c)** precipitations with tumor serum; supernatant from **(c)** precipitated with PAb122 medium **(d)**; first **(e)**, second **(f)**, and fourth **(g)** precipitations with PAb122 medium; supernatant from **(g)**, precipitated with tumor serum **(h)**. The tumor serum used for these precipitations did not bind p53 directly.

stable during storage at −20° C than the complexes in extracts from human or monkey cells as judged by immunoprecipitation of large T antigen with PAb122 antibody.

Preliminary results from two laboratories using PAb122 antibody suggest that the form of large T antigen involved in DNA binding may be different in SV40-infected and SV40-transformed monkey cells. In an investigation of *in vitro* DNA binding activity in extracts of SV40-transformed monkey cells, Carol Prives (*personal communication*) has found that PAb122 antibody precipitated a large fraction of the large T antigen able to bind to the origin of SV40 DNA. This suggests that much of the large T antigen able to bind specifically to SV40 DNA is complexed with p53 in these SV40-transformed cells. In contrast, Lois Tack (*personal communication*) obtained evidence that most of the large T antigen that is bound *in vivo* to replicating SV40 chromatin is not in complexes with p53. In her experiments, 80 to 90% of 90S 5 min pulse-labeled SV40 replicating chromatin from extracts of SVO-infected monkey cells were immunoprecipitated by SV40 tumor serum or a monoclonal antibody specific for large T antigen (PAb101, formerly called clone 412) (13), whereas PAb122 antibody precipitated only about 10% of the SV40 replicating chromatin.

The examples just cited of the analysis of p53 with monoclonal antibody PAb122 are quite preliminary and are intended to show that research on p53 is very active. Many questions about p53 and its interaction with other proteins remain unanswered. The use of monoclonal antibodies specific for p53 should play a part in elucidating the structure and function of this interesting cellular protein.

ACKNOWLEDGMENTS

I thank Robert Harrison and Susan Tamowski for excellent technical assistance, Frank O'Neill for cell lines, and Lionel Crawford for cells, radioimmunoassay probes, and helpful information. I appreciate the communication of unpublished results by Varda Rotter, Janet Butel, Carol Prives, and Lois Tack and the antibody analysis performed by Cliff Stocks and Seth Pincus. I am very grateful to Theodore Gurney, Jr., for encouragement and for critical reading of this manuscript and to Maurine Vaughan for expert typing. This work was supported by Public Health Service Research grant CA-21797 from the National Cancer Institute.

REFERENCES

1. Basilico, C., and Zouzias, D. (1976): Regulation of viral transcription and tumor antigen expression in cells transformed by simian virus 40. *Proc. Natl. Acad. Sci. USA*, 73:1931–1935.

2. Chandrasekaran, K., McFarland, V. W., Simmons, D. T., Dziadek, M., Gurney, E. G., and Mora, P. T. (1981): Quantitation and characterization of a species-specific and embryo-stage-dependent 55-kilodalton phosphoprotein also present in cells transformed by simian virus 40. *Proc. Natl. Acad. Sci. USA*, 78:6953–6957.

3. Chang, C., Simmons, D. T., Martin, M. A., and Mora, P. T. (1979): Identification and partial characterization of new antigens from simian virus 40-transformed mouse cells. *J. Virol.*, 31:463–471.

4. Crawford, L. V., Pim, D. C., Gurney, E. G., Goodfellow, P., and Taylor-Papadimitriou, J. (1981): Detection of a common feature in several human tumor cell lines: A 53,000-dalton protein. *Proc. Natl. Acad. Sci. USA*, 78:41–45.

5. DeLeo, A. B., Jay, G., Appella, E., Dubois, G. C., Law, L. W., and Old, L. J. (1979): Detection of a transformation-related antigen in chemically induced sarcomas and other transformed cells of the mouse. *Proc. Natl. Acad. Sci. USA*, 76:2420–2424.

6. Deppert, W., Gurney, E. G., and Harrison, R. O. (1981): Monoclonal antibodies against simian virus 40 tumor antigens: Analysis of antigenic binding sites using adenovirus type 2-simian virus 40 hybrid viruses. *J. Virol.*, 37:478–482.

7. Deppert, W., Hanke, K., and Henning, R. (1980): Simian virus 40 T-antigen-related cell surface antigen: Serological demonstration on simian virus 40-transformed monolayer cells *in situ*. *J. Virol.*, 35:505–518.

8. Dippold, W. G., Jay, G., DeLeo, A. B., Khoury, G., and Old, L. J. (1981): p53 transformation-related protein: Detection by monoclonal antibody in mouse and human cells. *Proc. Natl. Acad. Sci. USA*, 78:1695–1699.

9. Engvall, E., and Perlmann, P. (1972): Enzyme-linked immunosorbent assay, ELISA. III. Quantitation of specific antibodies by enzyme-labeled anti-immunoglobulin in antigen coated tubes. *J. Immunol.*, 109:129–135.

10. Fanning, E., Burger, C., and Gurney, E. G. (1981): Comparison of T antigen-associated host phosphoproteins from SV40-infected and -transformed cells of different species. *J. Gen. Virol.*, 55:367–378.

11. Galfrè, G., Howe, S. C., Milstein, C., Butcher, G. W., and Howard, J. C. (1977): Antibodies to major histocompatibility antigens produced by hybrid cell lines. *Nature*, 266:550–552.

12. Gurney, E. G., and Gurney, T., Jr. (1979): Density-dependent inhibition of both growth and T-antigen expression in revertants isolated from simian virus 40-transformed mouse SVT2 cells. *J. Virol.*, 32:661–671.

13. Gurney, E. G., Harrison, R. O., and Fenno, J. (1980): Monoclonal antibodies against simian virus 40 T antigens: Evidence for distinct subclasses of large T antigen and for similarities among nonviral T antigens. *J. Virol.*, 34:752–763.

14. Harlow, E., Crawford, L. V., Pim, D. C., and Williamson, N. M. (1981): Monoclonal antibodies specific for simian virus 40 tumor antigens. *J. Virol.*, 39:861–869.

15. Jay, G., Khoury, G., DeLeo, A. B., Dippold, W. G., and Old, L. J. (1981): p53 transformation-related protein: Detection of an associated phosphotransferase activity. *Proc. Natl. Acad. Sci. USA*, 78:2932–2936.

16. Köhler, G., and Milstein, C. (1975): Continuous cultures of fused cells secreting antibody of predefined specificity. *Nature*, 256:495–497.

17. Kress, M., May, E., Cassingena, R., and May, P. (1979): Simian virus 40-transformed cells express new species of proteins precipitable by anti-simian virus 40 tumor serum. *J. Virol.*, 31:472–483.

18. Lane, D. P., and Crawford, L. V. (1979): T antigen is bound to a host protein in SV40-transformed cells. *Nature*, 278:261–263.

19. Lane, D. P., and Robbins, A. K. (1978): An immunochemical investigation of SV40 T antigens. I. Production, properties, and specificity of a rabbit antibody to purified simian virus 40 large-T antigen. *Virology*, 87:182–193.

20. Linzer, D. I. H., and Levine, A. J. (1979): Characterization of a 54K dalton cellular SV40 tumor antigen present in SV40-transformed cells and uninfected embryonal carcinoma cells. *Cell*, 17:43–52.

21. Linzer, D. I. H., Maltzman, W., and Levine, A. J. (1979): The SV40 A gene product is required for the production of a 54,000 MW cellular tumor antigen. *Virology*, 98:308–318.

22. McCormick, F., and Harlow, E. (1980): Association of a murine 53,000-dalton phosphoprotein with simian virus 40 large-T antigen in transformed cells. *J. Virol.*, 34:213–224.

23. Mora, P. T., Chandrasekaran, K., and McFarland, V. M. (1980): An embryo protein induced by SV40 virus transformation of mouse cells. *Nature*, 288:722–724.

24. O'Neill, F. J. (1975): Control of nuclear division in SV40 and adenovirus type 12 transformed mouse 3T3 cells. *Int. J. Cancer*, 15:715–723.

25. Oren, M., Maltzman, W., and Levine, A. J. (1981): Post-translational regulation of the 54K cellular tumor antigen in normal and transformed cells. *Mol. Cell. Biol.*, 1:101–110.

26. Rotter, V., Witte, O. N., Coffman, R., and Baltimore, D. (1980): Abelson murine leukemia virus-induced tumors elicit antibodies against a host cell protein, p50. *J. Virol.*, 36:547–555.

27. Simmons, D. T. (1980): Characterization of tau antigens isolated from uninfected and simian virus 40-infected monkey cells and papovavirus-transformed cells. *J. Virol.*, 36:519–525.

28. Smith, A. E., Smith, R., and Paucha, E. (1979): Characterization of different tumor antigens present in cells transformed by simian virus 40. *Cell*, 18:335–346.

29. Soule, H. R., Lanford, R. E., and Butel, J. S. (1980): Antigenic and im-
    munogenic characteristics of nuclear and membrane-associated simian virus
    40 tumor antigen. *J. Virol.*, 33:887–901.
30. Voller, A., Bidwell, D. E., and Bartlett, A. (1976): Enzyme immunoassays
    in diagnostic medicine theory and practice. *Bull. WHO*, 53:55–65.

Advances in Viral Oncology, Volume 2, edited by
George Klein. Raven Press, New York © 1982.

Control of Cellular Levels of the Transformation-Associated 53–55 K Proteins (p53s)

Pierre May, Evelyne May, and *Michel Kress

Institute for Cancer Research, 94802 Villejuif Cedex, France

In addition to the virus-coded large T and small T antigens, cell-coded proteins with a molecular weight of about 53,000 to 55,000 can be immunoprecipitated from extracts of the cells infected or transformed by SV40 using anti-SV40 tumor serum (3,5,8–11,13–15,19,21–24,32,34,35,37,46–48). These proteins have been referred to as p53. Similar p53 components were detected in relatively high amounts in mouse embryonal carcinoma, in mouse tumor cell lines transformed by different agents, and in low amounts in certain normal mouse or monkey cells (14,15,23,24,46). Comparable p53 was also found in high amounts in malignant cultured human cells (7,9,46). Expression of p53 in some rapidly dividing normal human cells, was shown to correlate with the growth characteristics of the culture: cells in the proliferative phase contained high levels of p53, whereas contact-inhibited cells contained little or no p53 (9). It was also observed that p53 is detectable in mouse lymphocytes following mitogenic stimulation, but not in nondividing lymphocytes (39,40). Recently, it was reported that primary cells from midgestation mouse, hamster, or rat embryos all contain high levels of p53 (4,41).

The expression of p53 was extensively studied in cells infected or transformed by SV40. These studies have greatly contributed to our knowledge of some regulatory mechanisms for the expression

*Present address: National Cancer Institute, National Institutes of Health, Bethesda, Maryland 20014

of p53. It was demonstrated that p53s form a complex with the nuclear SV40 large T antigen (15,22,36,37) and that the formation of this complex results in a stabilization of p53s and, consequently, in a considerable increase in cellular levels of p53s.

This article will attempt to summarize recent information on the control of p53 expression in mammalian cells. The field of SV40-transformed or infected cells will be briefly reviewed, with particular emphasis on some results obtained in our laboratory. In addition, certain lines of investigation on some other cell systems or situations will also be described.

EXPRESSION OF p53 IN CELLS INFECTED OR TRANSFORMED BY SV40

Association of p53 with SV40 Large T Antigen

Lane and Crawford (22) were the first to find that antisera specific for SV40 large T antigen were able coordinately to precipitate SV40 large T antigen and p53 from extracts of SV40-transformed mouse cells, although the antisera used were unable to recognize p53 directly; this observation led the authors to conclude that p53 occurs in a complex with large T antigen in SV40-transformed mouse cells. Consistent with this conclusion, sucrose gradient analysis of extracts of mouse transformed cells showed that the p53 component and a fraction of the large T antigen sediment together at about 14 to 16 S. A number of similar observations were then reported on the binding of p53 to large T antigen in SV40-infected or -transformed cells of mouse, hamster, rabbit, and human origin (7,11,13,19,32). It was reported that the association of large T and p53 must involve noncovalent bonds (37) and that p53 usually is found in the nucleus (9,14,35,37). The formation of a similar complex between SV40 large T antigen and p53 in SV40-infected CV1 monkey cells was also demonstrated (15). It was similarly shown that in Epstein-Barr virus (EBV)-transformed cells, p53 components were complexed with EBV-determined nuclear antigen (EBNA) (25). Recently,

McCormick et al. (37) showed that addition of purified D2 protein (biologically equivalent to SV40 large T antigen) or of purified large T antigen from SV80 cells to lysates of labeled embryonal carcinoma cells, followed by a 15-min incubation at room temperature, resulted in the binding of D2 or large T antigen to p53. The entire p53 component detected in these lysates was able to bind to added T antigen, whereas no other cellular protein appeared to form a stable complex with T antigen under these conditions.

Early studies (22,32) showed that large T antigen and p53, when synthesized *in vitro* in the same translation mixture, did not form a complex (Fig. 1). Considering the results of McCormick et al. (37), it appears very likely that the inability of large T antigen and p53 produced by *in vitro* translation to form a complex reflects the requirement of some posttranslational modifications of large T antigen and/or p53 in order for the complex to be formed. A good candidate for such posttranscriptional modification(s) is the phosphorylation of large T antigen, since it has been consistently observed that the p53-associated form of large T antigen is more highly phosphorylated than the free form (11,13,37). This should not, however, be construed to mean that other posttranslational modifications of large T antigen and/or p53 are not required for the formation of large T-p53 complex.

Immunological and Structural Relationship Between Various p53s

One of the first questions raised by the discovery of p53 components in SV40-transformed cells was whether these components were host cell- or virus-coded. We now know that they are host cell-coded, since a considerable body of evidence has accumulated which shows that both immunologically and structurally related p53 components can be detected in mouse cells that are free of any SV40 contamination as well as in cells originating from a variety of animal species. It is noteworthy, however, that some of the first indications for the host cell origin of p53s in SV40-transformed cells were the

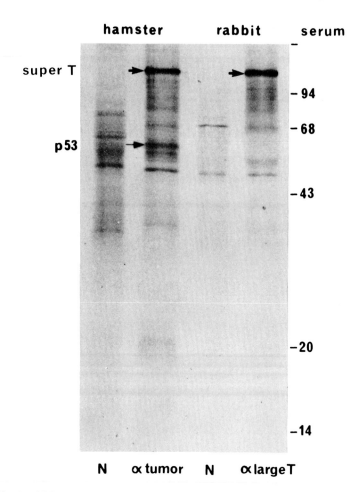

FIG. 1. SDS polyacrylamide gel autoradiogram showing that T antigen and p53 do not form a complex when they are synthesized *in vitro*. Samples of both preparations of RNA specifying T antigen and p53, respectively, were mixed. The mixture was translated *in vitro* and the translation products were immunoprecipitated with hamster anti-SV40 tumor serum (α tumor) (containing some antibodies specific for T antigen and some specific for p53), rabbit anti serum directed against large T antigen (α large T), and normal hamster (or rabbit) serum *(N)*. Immunoprecipitated proteins were resolved by 12.5% SDS polyacrylamide gel electrophoresis and visualized by auto-radiography. In this experiment, T antigen mRNA was actually coding for 115 K super T antigen. This super T antigen, when synthesized *in vivo*, was shown to form stable complex with *in vivo* synthesized p53. Notice that the rabbit α large T serum immu-noprecipitates super T but it does not coimmunoprecipitate p53, as it would do if *in vitro* synthesized p53 and super T complex to one another, whereas the hamster α tumor serum containing specific antibodies for both super T and p53 does immuno-precipitate both proteins. (From May et al., ref. 33.)

following: (a) the methionine-labeled tryptic digests of p53s and SV40 large T antigen did not share any common tryptic peptide, and (b) the mRNAs coding for p53s did not contain any detectable viral sequence (21,32,48). The p53 components detected in the various mammalian species share common antigenic determinant(s) since specific monoclonal antibodies to mouse p53 were found to react with p53s in the cells of other mammalian species (7,9,14,15,45). The structures of p53s from various mammalian species also appeared to be partially related when tested by tryptic peptide mapping or by partial proteolysis digest (34,46,47). Studies were performed on the structural relationship between the p53s detected in various cell lines transformed by different agents but originating from a same animal species. Thus, hamster cells transformed by various primate papovaviruses (simian virus 40, BK virus, and JC virus) were shown to synthesize indistinguishable p53, as determined by two-dimensional peptide mapping (46). Cell lines derived from spontaneous human tumors contain p53s very similar to the p53 from SV80 cells, as judged by partial proteolysis patterns (7).

A comparison of fingerprints of p53s detected in SV40- and nonviral-transformed mouse cells was performed by Maltzman et al. (27). The chromobead elution patterns of methionine-labeled tryptic peptides of the mouse p53s, derived from embryonal carcinoma cells, 3T12 cells, and chemically transformed cells, were all similar or identical. The p53 component synthesized by *in vitro* translation of mRNA from SV40-transformed cells also produced a polypeptide with similar or identical methionine-labeled tryptic peptides. The p53s from all of these diverse sources appeared to be closely related or identical, and they had eight methionine-labeled tryptic peptides in common with the p53 obtained after *in vivo* labeling of SV40-transformed cell lines. However, the p53 derived from SV40-transformed cells labeled *in vivo* produced three to five additional methionine-labeled tryptic peptides that were not detected in the other cell lines or with the p53 component synthesized by *in vitro* translation. Maltzman et al. (27) suggested that these additional peptides could be the result of a posttranslational modification of the mouse p53 component that is specific to SV40-transformed cells.

However, phosphorylation does not seem to be involved in that modification step, as shown by a chromobead elution pattern of the mixture of a digest of ^{32}PO$_4$-labeled p53 from SV40-transformed mouse cell line SVT2 with a ^{35}S methionine-labeled tryptic digest of the same protein (27).

In a similar manner, we studied the rat p53s obtained either *in vivo* or *in vitro* from the SV40-transformed V11F1 clone 1 subclone 7 rat cells (hereafter called subclone 7 cells). We compared the two-dimensional fingerprints of methionine-containing tryptic peptides of the p53 derived from subclone 7 cells labeled *in vivo* with (^{35}S)methionine with those of the p53 component synthesized by *in vitro* translation of mRNA obtained from these same subclone 7 cells. The results (Fig.2) show that the tryptic peptides of both rat p53 components are virtually identical, except for the peptide lacking in the fingerprints of *in vitro* synthesized p53. This observation, as well as that of Maltzman et al. (27), could be related to the above-mentioned observation that posttranslational modifications of SV40 large T antigen and/or p53 appear to be required for the formation of the large T-p53 complex.

SV40 Large T Antigen Is Involved in the Expression of High Levels of p53

In 1979, Linzer et al. (24) reported that infection or transformation of 3T3 cells by SV40 wild type resulted in a 25- to 50-fold increase in the cellular level of p53, compared to that of control 3T3 cells. However, temperature-sensitive *A* gene mutants of SV40, at the nonpermissive temperature, failed to initiate the maximal increased levels of p53 observed in virus-infected or -transformed cells. Recently, Oren et al. (42) observed that 3T3 and SV40-transformed 3T3 cells (SV3T3) contain about the same levels of mRNA coding for p53, as tested by *in vitro* translation experiments, whereas SV3T3 cells contain significantly higher levels of p53 than control 3T3 cells, as observed by *in vivo* labeling of proteins and immunoprecipitation. These authors deduced from these results that p53 is much more stable in SV3T3 cells than in 3T3 cells and this suggestion

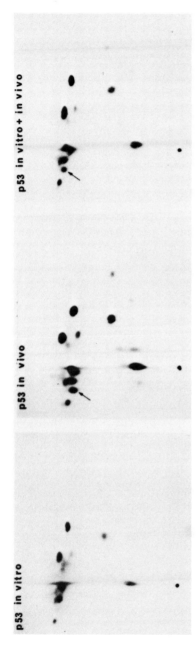

FIG. 2. Comparison of (^{35}S) methionine-labeled tryptic peptides synthesized **(middle)** *in vivo* by subclone 7 cells or **(left)** by *in vitro* translation of mRNA specifying p53 from the same cells. **Middle:** Subclone 7 cell cultures were labeled for 3 hr with (^{35}S) methionine. After labeling, the proteins were extracted and immunoprecipitated with anti-SV40 tumor serum. P53 component was separated by SDS polyacrylamide gel electrophoresis of the immunoprecipitated proteins and then eluted from the appropriate gel slice. Conditions for radiolabeling and extraction of cells, immunoprecipitation and electrophoresis of labeled proteins, and elution of labeled p53 from polyacrylamide gels have been described (21). **Left:** A preparation of p53 mRNA was obtained by fractionating polyadenylated cytoplasmic RNA from subclone 7 cells through sucrose density gradient. The RNA from each fraction was ethanol-precipitated and then redissolved in H_2O. The reticulocyte lysate system containing (^{35}S) methionine was programmed with the RNA from each fraction; the translation products were immunoprecipitated with anti-SV40 tumor serum. The sucrose gradient fractionation had been shown to enable us to separate the 17 S mRNA specifying p53 from the other size classes of mRNAs (32). The procedures for preparation of polyadenylated cytoplasmic RNA, sucrose gradient fractionation, *in vitro* translation in reticulocyte lysate, immunoprecipitation and analysis of labeled proteins by SDS-PAGE, and elution of labeled p53 from polyacrylamide gel have been described (21,32). After elution, the p53s synthesized *in vivo* or *in vitro* were precipitated, oxidized with performic acid, treated with trypsin, and analyzed by two-dimensional separation on thin-layer plates as described (29). Electrophoresis at pH 4.7 was in the horizontal dimension, with the origin on the left and the cathode on the right. Ascending chromatography was in the vertical dimension. (^{35}S) methionine-labeled tryptic peptides were visualized by fluorography (2). **Right:** A peptide map of an equal mixture of both *in vivo* and *in vitro* synthesized p53 components. *Arrow* indicates the peptide that is lacking in the fingerprints of *in vitro* synthesized p53.

was confirmed by pulse-chase analysis of p53 in 3T3 and SV3T3 cells. In addition, since the extreme stability of p53 appears to be a thermo-sensitive characteristic of cells transformed by a SV40 *tsA* mutant, it was concluded that a functional large T antigen was required to provide high levels of p53 *in vivo*, with the stabilizing effect of large T antigen being exerted through the formation of the large T-p53 complex (42). In the next section, we will report some experiments that have relevance to the question of which function of large T antigen is involved in the control of p53 expression.

The Study of SV40 115 K Super T Antigen as an Approach to Dissociating Different Functions of SV40 Large T Antigen

It has recently become clear that the role of *A* gene in DNA replication is distinct from its role in transformation. In 1977, Gluzman et al. (12) isolated permissive transformed monkey cells that displayed the SV40 large T antigen, but failed to support the replication of SV40 *tsA* mutants at the nonpermissive temperature. To account for this, the authors have suggested that the gene *A* product has separate functions for transformation and initiation of viral DNA synthesis, and only the former function is expressed in the transformed permissive monkey cells. Additional evidence that the role of the *A* gene in DNA replication is distinct from its role in transformation comes from the properties of two temperature-sensitive mutants of SV40, *tsA* 1499 (43) and *tsA* 1642 (6), and from the biological properties of SV40 115 K super T antigen from SV40-transformed V11F1 clone 1 subclone 7 cells (30). Mutant *tsA* 1499 lacks 81 base pairs around 0.21 map unit and is heat sensitive for lytic growth and cold sensitive for transformation. Mutant *tsA* 1642 corresponds to a single nucleotide substitution at position 3379, according to the nucleotide numbering of Reddy et al. (44). At nonpermissive temperature in the lytic cycle *tsA* 1642 accumulates viral DNA, T antigens, and late proteins at near wild-type levels, but produces only low levels of infectious virus. On the other hand, *tsA* 1642 is markedly defective in transformation.

Recently, May et al. (30) similarly observed the dissociation of the role of SV40 large T antigen in DNA replication and its role in transformation by studying the biological properties of 115 K super T expressed in an SV40-transformed rat cell line. This study showed that super T antigen, although unable to induce the initiation of SV40 DNA replication efficiently, is indeed able to induce cell transformation and to enhance the cellular level of p53. These data are reported in the following subsections.

Construction of a Recombinant Cosmid SVE 5 Kb Carrying the Gene for 115 K Super T Antigen

Multiple species of T antigens with molecular weight distinct from normal-sized large T antigen can be identified in a variety of SV40-transformed rat and mouse cell lines. Species of T antigen with a molecular weight considerably larger than that of normal-sized large T antigen are referred to as super T antigens (21). As already reported, SV40-transformed rat cell line V11F1 clone 1 subclone 7 produces a single species of super T antigen of 115,000 M_r in the absence of detectable traces of large T antigen (86,000 M_r) (32). We have previously shown that this super T antigen (super T) is an elongated form of large T antigen, which contains a duplication of that part of large T antigen corresponding to the genome portion extending approximately from 0.46 to 0.35 map units, as determined by fingerprint analysis of super T and by S1 mapping analysis of 115 K super T mRNA (29). Moreover, the arrangement of SV40-integrated DNA sequences of subclone 7 cells was established by using Southern blot hybridization and by sequencing cloned restriction fragments (28). It was thus shown that the sequence duplication in 115 K super T mRNA is a consequence of a homologous duplication of a 573 nucleotide sequence in the viral DNA integrated in subclone 7 cells. In addition, this analysis reveals that the two copies of the 573 nucleotide repeated sequence bracket a 93 nucleotide sequence that is a nearly perfect, inverted repeat of a viral segment located farther than 1,200 nucleotides upstream in the early viral region (Fig. 3). In the course of the latter study, a

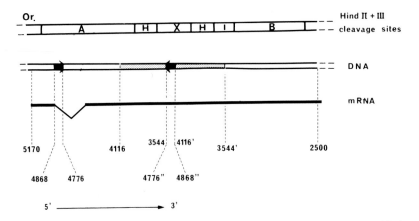

FIG. 3. Diagrammatic representation of the super T gene configuration. **Top:** Hind II + III restriction map of super T gene. By comparing with the familiar map of authentic SV40 DNA it should be noted that fragment H is duplicated, the two copies separated by a new fragment x. **Middle:** Locations and sizes of direct duplication *(stippled area)* and 93 bp repeats *(solid block)* whose orientation is indicated by the *arrowheads.* **Bottom:** The super T mRNA. *Caret* indicates that segment known to be spliced out during the maturation of large T mRNA and by analogy probably spliced out in the maturation of super T mRNA. The numbers refer to nucleotide numbers (28). Nucleotide numbers of downstream direct repeat unit are marked with *single quotes* and nucleotide numbers of the downstream inverted repeat are marked with *double quotes.* (From May et al., ref. 28.)

5kb fragment containing the entire gene coding for 115 K super T antigen was cloned into the cosmid pHC 79 resulting in a recombinant cosmid SVE 5kb. This hybrid cosmid was used to study the biological properties of 115 K super T antigen.

Transformation of Rat Cells with SVE 5kb

The transforming activity of the viral sequence in SVE 5kb was tested by transfecting secondary cultures of rat kidney cells , using the calcium phosphate technique (49) and quantifying dense foci overgrowing the normal monolayers. Dishes were scored for foci after 3 to 4 weeks of incubation. We used as a control the recombinant plasmid pSV1 containing pBR322 and the early SV40 genes (1). In repeated assays, the transformation efficiency was approximately 50% that of the control plasmid (30).

Low Efficiency of SVE 5kb DNA in
Complementing *tsA* 58 DNA

The capacity of SVE 5kb DNA to complement *tsA* 58 DNA at nonpermissive temperature (41°C) was tested by cotransfecting CV1 cells (100 mm plates) with SV40 *tsA* 58 DNA (0.1 μg/plate) and SVE 5kb (0.1μg/plate), using the DEAE-dextran procedure (38). Cells amplifying SV40 DNA were detected *in situ* 44 hr after transfection, by the rapid method described by Hayday et al. (16). Briefly, the SV40-infected CV1 cells were transferred to nitrocellulose filters and their DNA was immobilized *in situ*. The filters were exposed to a nick-translated probe of SV40 DNA and only those cells containing multiple copies of SV40 DNA showed detectable hybridization. The extent of hybridization was monitored by autoradiography. Comparison was made with several parallel sets of CV1 cell cultures cotransfected with *tsA* 58 DNA and with serial dilutions of pSV1 recombinant plasmid, respectively. It was observed that the hybrid cosmid SVE 5kb (containing the gene coding for 115 K super T) was approximately 100-fold less efficient in complementing *tsA* 58 DNA at nonpermissive temperature than the hybrid plasmid pSV1. It should be noted that both recombinant DNA pSV1 and SVE 5kb contain pBR322 DNA sequences, including the "poison" sequences (26). Taken together, these experiments show that 115 K super T antigen is relatively efficient in inducing transformation of rat or mouse cells, but poorly efficient in initiating SV40 DNA replication.

High Levels of p53 in SVE 5kb-Transformed Cell Lines

Cell lines derived from foci induced either by SVE 5kb or by pSV1 were compared for their relative levels of p53 component. The cell lines were tested as early as their second subcultures. The SVE 5kb-transformed cells regularly contain relative amounts of p53 of the same order as those of the pSV1-transformed cells. This comparison was made by densitometry of autoradiograms of gels such as that of Fig. 4.

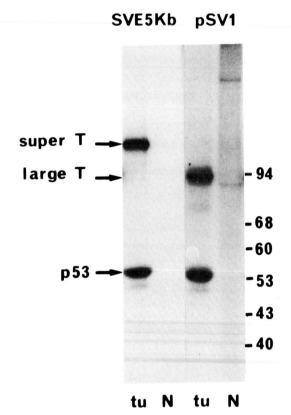

FIG. 4. Autoradiogram showing high levels of p53 in rat cells transformed by the hybrid cosmid SVE 5 Kb carrying the gene for super T. SVE 5 Kb- and pSV1-transformed rat cells were seeded (5 × 10⁵ cells per 10 cm petri dish, at their third and sixth subcultures, respectively) and grown in Eagle minimal essential medium supplemented with 10% fetal calf serum. Six days after seeding, the cultures were labeled for 3 hr with ^{32}PO₄. After labeling, the proteins were extracted from the cells and immunoprecipitated either by normal hamster serum *(N)* or by anti-SV40 tumor serum (*tu*). The immunoprecipitates were analyzed on a 7.5% SDS polyacrylamide gel. After staining and drying, the gels were processed for autoradiography. The procedures for extraction of cells and for immunoprecipitation, electrophoresis, and autoradiography were described (21). The numbers at the right of the gel indicate the positions of the molecular-weight markers ($M_r × 10^{-3}$). The recombinant DNAs used to transform the cell lines are indicated above each track.

This observation, made soon after the establishment of transformation, suggests that super T antigen is able to induce the production of high levels of p53 in SVE 5kb-transformed cells.

Comparison of the Affinities of p53 for 115 K Super T and Large T Antigens

The following experiment was performed to compare the affinities of p53 for 115 K super and large T antigens, respectively. We examined a rat cell line V11F1 clone 1 subclone 4, a sister of subclone 7, which exhibited a progressive change in the mobility pattern of proteins immunoprecipitable with anti-SV40 tumor serum (Fig. 5). Whereas early passages (10 to 20) contained few if any detectable 115 K super-T antigen molecules, the later passages (40 to 100) contained progressively increasing amounts of 115 K super T antigen. It has recently been shown that heterogeneity of subclone 4 results from rearrangements of the viral sequence after the initial integration of SV40 into the cell DNA (E. May, *in preparation*). Later passages of subclone 4 consisted of two populations of SV40-transformed rat cells: one expressing large T antigen, and the other expressing 115 K super T antigen, the latter population progressively overgrowing the former. Cultures of subclone 4 cells (passage 103) were labeled with $^{32}PO_4$. After labeling, a sample of extracts from the cell nuclei was centrifuged through 5 to 20% sucrose density gradient in PBS containing 2.5 M KCl. Aliquots of the individually collected fractions were immunoprecipitated with anti-SV40 tumor serum and then subjected to SDS polyacrylamide electrophoresis (Fig. 6). Large T antigen appears to sediment mainly as a free form in fractions 3 and 4 (at about 5 S) whereas the majority of super T antigen is distributed between fractions 7 and 13 with maximum amounts in fractions 9 and 10 (approximately 15 S). A small proportion of super T antigen is detected in fraction 4 and 5 and might correspond to a free form of super T antigen. Moreover, the p53 component appears to sediment together with super T antigen. Taken

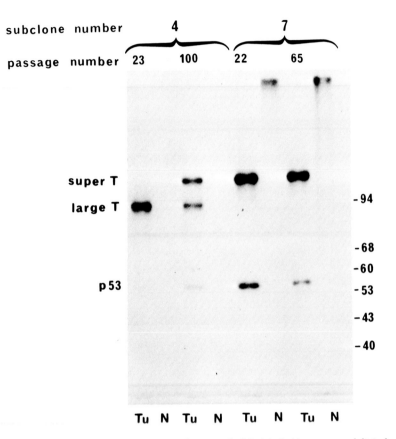

subclone number   4   7

passage number   23   100   22   65

super T

large T   - 94

- 68

- 60

p 53   - 53

- 43

- 40

Tu   N   Tu   N   Tu   N   Tu   N

FIG. 5. SDS polyacrylamide gel autoradiogram of $^{32}PO_4$-labeled immunoprecipitated proteins from extracts of subclones 4 and 7 derived from the V11F1 clone 1 rat cell line. Cultures of subclones 4 and 7, taken at various passages, were labeled with $^{32}PO_4$. After labeling, the proteins were extracted from the cells and reacted with normal hamster *(N)* and anti SV40 tumor *(Tu)* serum. The immunoprecipitates were analyzed on 7.5% SDS polyacrylamide gels; after staining and drying, the gels were processed for autoradiography. The procedures for radiolabeling and extraction of cells and for immunoprecipitation, electrophoresis, and autoradiography have been described (21). The numbers at the right of the gel indicate the position of molecular weight markers ($M_r \times 10^{-3}$).

together, these observations strongly suggest that in the nuclear extracts from subclone 4 at passage 103, p53 is bound to 115 K super T antigen, forming a rapidly sedimenting complex, whereas large T antigen exists in a free form, implying that p53 possesses a higher affinity for super T antigen than for large T antigen. The high affinity of p53 for 115 K super T antigen may explain the ability of 115 K super T antigen to induce high levels of p53 in SVE 5kb-transformed rat cells.

The properties of 115 K super T antigen, viewed as a whole, lead us to infer that transforming activity, rather than lytic activity, is the function of large T antigen, which is required for the expression of high levels of p53. Our results also suggest that when a large T gene is subjected to evolutionary changes, those variants that lose the ability to bind to p53 and to enhance p53 level are at selective disadvantage.

A BRIEF SURVEY OF THE CELL CONDITIONS IN WHICH HIGH LEVELS OF p53 ARE EXPRESSED

As a first approach to explaining the role of p53, it is interesting to note that all the cells expressing p53 appear to be characterized by a high mitotic activity. This important point emerges from a brief survey of the cell types or cellular states in which high levels of p53 are expressed.

1. Transformed cells or tumor cells were shown to contain high levels of p53; this point was well documented in the case of human and mouse cells (7–9,19,22).

2. Mouse or monkey cells infected with SV40 also contain detectable amounts of p53 (3,15,22,24,34,35,46); it is known that in these cells the expression of early viral region is rapidly followed by a mitogenic reaction of the host cells (17,20,31,33).

3. In certain cultured normal human cells, such as rapidly dividing kidney epithelium cells and cells derived from fetal brain, p53 was detected, but it was found predominantly or exclusively in those cells that were in the proliferative phase (9).

4. Milner and McCormick (39) reported that p53 could not be detected in nondividing lymphocytes, but this protein was induced when the same cells entered the division cycle in response to concanavalin A treatment. The induction of p53 was shown to occur

within 4 hr after the addition of concanavalin A, coinciding with the commitment of cells to enter the division cycle. This observation suggested a role for p53 during the transition from Go into the division cycle (40). Moreover, these authors reported that induction of p53 was prevented when the cells were treated with α-amanitin during the first 3 hr of concanavalin A stimulation, suggesting a possible control of p53 expression at the level of gene transcription (40).

5. Jay et al. (18) detected p53 in normal mouse thymocytes, which might be explained by the extremely high mitotic rate characteristic of a subpopulation of thymocytes.

6. Recently, Mora and his colleagues (4,41) found relatively high levels of p53 in primary cells from midgestation mouse, hamster, or rat embryos. This could reflect the fact that certain primary cells of midgestation murine embryo might be characterized either by a capacity to constitutively express the p53 component, or by an intensive mitotic activity.

FIG. 6. Sucrose gradient centrifugation of nuclear extracts from V11F1 clone 1 subclone 4 cells. V11F1 clone 1 subclone 4 cell cultures (passage 103) in 10 cm petri dishes were labeled for 3 hr with $^{32}PO_4$. After labeling, the cultures were washed with phosphate buffered saline (PBS), then 0.5 ml/petri dish of 0.1% Tween 80 was added and left for 5 min. Three ml/dish of ice cold isotonic buffer (IB) (0.25 M sucrose, 10m M triethanolamine, pH7, 25m M NaCl, 5m M MgCl$_2$) was then added. The nuclei were pelleted at 3,000 rpm for 5 min, washed with IB, and lysed in NaCl 0.5 M (1 ml/10 petri dishes). The suspension obtained was centrifuged at 10,000 rpm for 30 min. The supernatant was dialyzed overnight against ice-cold PBS and recentrifuged in order to be clarified. The last supernatant was made 2.5 M in KCl; 0.5 ml of this supernatant was layered on 5 to 20% 12 ml sucrose gradient in PBS-2.5 M KCl. After the gradient was centrifuged at 31,000 rpm in an SW 41 rotor for 18 hr at 4°C, it was fractionated. Individual fractions were twofold diluted with H^{2}O, and then immunoprecipitated with anti SV40 tumor serum and analyzed by 7.5% SDS polyacrylamide gel electrophoresis. Fractions 3 and 7correspond to the positions of bovine serum albumin (4-5 S) and active bovine liver catalase (11-12 S) respectively, sedimented in a parallel gradient. The procedures for radiolabeling of cells and immunoprecipitation and electrophoresis of labeled proteins have been described (21). The fraction numbers are indicated below each track. The numbers at the right of the gels indicate the positions of the molecular-weight markers (M$_r$ × 10^{-3}).

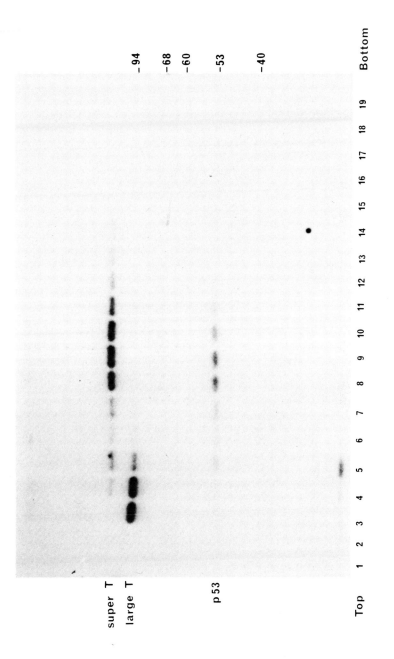

CONCLUSION

This brief survey suggests that p53 is involved in the control of cell growth, since p53 expression usually appears as a feature of cells characterized by a high mitotic activity. However, it is convenient to make a distinction between three types of situations in which this occurs:

1. In rapidly dividing cells, such as normal human kidney epithelium, elevated levels of p53 were found only during the proliferative phase, whereas little or no p53 was detected in contact-inhibited cells (9). This suggests that in normal cells a transient increase in the p53 level might be required at a specific point in the cell cycle to allow further progression through the cell cycle.

2. In the case of resting lymphocytes stimulated to enter the mitotic cell cycle by concanavalin A, the timing of p53 appearance after the addition of concanavalin A suggested a role for this protein during transition from Go into the division cycle (40). However, high levels of p53 were observed during the progression of the cells through all of the cell cycle.

3. In cells either transformed or derived from tumors, expression of elevated levels of p53 is generally constitutive. The most documented model system in this field is SV40-transformed cell lines. The steady state high levels of p53 in SV40-transformed cells result from a considerable increase in p53 half-life mediated by the formation of large T-p53 complex (22,42). It is likely that persistent expression of high levels of p53 could provoke a disruption in the normal control of cell division and thereby contribute to some growth characteristics of the transformed phenotype. It is noteworthy that the transforming function rather than the lytic function of SV40 large T antigen appears to correlate with the capacity of large T antigen to induce high levels of p53 in SV40-transformed cells (30).

A number of questions might now be raised. At what specific point in the cell cycle does a transient increase occur in the p53 level? Does p53 act as a controlling signal? How is the expression of p53 temporally regulated during the normal cell cycle? In cells transformed by agents other than SV40, is it possible to identify proteins able to form a stable complex with p53 components? Whether p53 is involved in embryonic differentiation and development is also open to question. It seems very likely that all or most of these questions will be answered in the near future.

ACKNOWLEDGMENTS

We thank L. Daya-Grosjean and M. Poritz for critical comments and P. T. Mora for providing us with information in advance of publication. This work was supported by grant 60803665 from the Centre National de la Recherche Scientifique.

REFERENCES

1. Benoist, C., and Chambon, P. (1980): Deletions covering the putative promoter region of early mRNAs of simian virus 40 do not abolish T-antigen expression. *Proc. Natl. Acad. Sci. USA*, 77:3865–3869.
2. Bonner, W. M., and Stedman, J. D. (1978): Efficient fluorography of ^{3}H and ^{14}C on thin layers. *Anal. Biochem.*, 89:247–256.
3. Carroll, R. B., Muello, K., and Melero, J. A. (1980): Coordinate expression of the 48 K host nuclear phosphoprotein and SV40 T Ag upon primary infection of mouse cells. *Virology*, 102:447–452.
4. Chandrasekaran, K., McFarland, V. W., Simmons, D. T., Dziadek, M., Gurney, E. G., and Mora, P. T. (1981): Quantitation and characterization of a species specific and embryo age dependent 55 K MW phosphoprotein which is also present in cells transformed by SV40. *Proc. Natl. Acad. Sci. USA*, 78:6953–6957.
5. Chang, C., Simmons, D. T., Martin, M. A., and Mora, P. T. (1979): Identification and partial characterization of new antigens from simian virus 40-transformed mouse cells. *J. Virol.*, 31:463–471.
6. Cosman, D. J., and Tevethia, M. J. (1981): Characterization of a temperature-sensitive, DNA-positive, non transforming mutant of simian virus 40. *Virology*, 112:605–624.
7. Crawford, L. V., Pim, D. C., Gurney, E. G., Goodfellow, P., and Taylor-Papadimitriou, J. (1981): Detection of a common feature in several human tumor cell lines. A 53,000-dalton protein. *Proc. Natl. Acad. Sci. USA*, 78:41–45.
8. DeLeo, A. B., Jay, G., Appella, E., Dubois, G. C., Law, L. W., and Old, L. J. (1979): Detection of a transformation related antigen in chemically induced sarcomas and other transformed cells of the mouse. *Proc. Natl. Acad. Sci. USA*, 76:2420–2424.

9. Dippold, W., Jay, G., Deleo, A. B., Khoury, G., and Old, L. J. (1981): p53 transformation-related protein: Detection by monoclonal antibody in mouse and human cells. *Proc. Natl. Acad. Sci. USA*, 78:1695–1699.

10. Edwards, C. A. F., Khoury, G., and Martin, R. G. (1979): Phosphorylation of T-antigen and control of T antigen expression in cells transformed by wild-type and tsA mutants of simian virus 40. *J. Virol.*, 29:753–762.

11. Fanning, E., Nowak, B., and Burger, C. (1981): Detection and characterization of multiple forms of simian virus 40 large T antigen. *J. Virol.*, 37:92–102.

12. Gluzman, Y., Davison, J., Oren, M., and Winocour, E. (1977): Properties of permissive monkey cells transformed by UV-irradiated simian virus 40. *J. Virol.*, 22:256–266.

13. Greenspan, D. S., and Carroll, R. B. (1981): Complex of simian virus 40 large tumor antigen and 48,000-dalton host tumor antigen. *Proc. Natl. Acad. Sci. USA*, 78:105–109.

14. Gurney, E. G., Harrison, R. O., and Fenno, J. (1980): Monoclonal antibodies against simian virus 40 T antigens: Evidence for distinct subclasses of large T antigen and for similarities among nonviral T antigens. *J. Virol.*, 34:752–763.

15. Harlow, E., Pim, D. C., and Crawford, L. V. (1981): Complex of simian virus 40 large-T antigen and host 53,000-molecular weight protein monkey cells. *J. Virol.*, 37:564–573.

16. Hayday, A., Gandini-Attardi, D., and Fried, M. (1981): Detection in situ of foreign DNA in eukaryotic cells. *Gene*, 15:53–65.

17. Hiscott, J. B., and Defendi, V. (1981): Simian virus gene A regulation of cellular DNA synthesis. II. In nonpermissive cells. *J. Virol.*, 37:802–812.

18. Jay, G., Deleo, A. B., Appella, E., Dubois, G. C., Law, L. W., Khoury, G., and Old, L. J. (1979): A common protein in murine sarcomas and leukemias. *Cold Spring Harbor Symp. Quant. Biol.*, 44:659–664.

19. Jay, G., Khoury, G., DeLeo, A. B., Dippold, W. G., and Old, L. J. (1981): p53 transformation-related protein: Detection of an associated phosphotransferase activity. *Proc. Natl. Acad. Sci. USA*, 78:2932–2936.

20. Khandjian, E. W., Matter, J. M., Leonard, N., and Weil, R. (1980): Simian virus 40 and polyoma virus stimulate overall cellular RNA and protein synthesis. *Proc. Natl. Acad. Sci. USA*, 77:1476–1480.

21. Kress, M., May, E., Cassingena, R., and May, P. (1979): Simian virus 40-transformed cells express new species of proteins precipitable by antisimian virus 40 tumor serum. *J. Virol.*, 31:472–483.

22. Lane, D. P., and Crawford, L. V. (1979): T antigen is bound to a host protein in SV40-transformed cells. *Nature*, 278:261–263.

23. Linzer, D. I. H., and Levine, A. J. (1979): Characterization of a 54 K dalton cellular SV40 tumor antigen present in SV40-transformed cells and uninfected embryonal carcinoma cells. *Cell*, 17:43–52.

24. Linzer, D. I. H., Maltzman, W., and Levine, A. J. (1979): The SV40 A gene product is required for the production of a 54,000 MW cellular tumor antigen. *Virology*, 98:308–318.

25. Luka, J., Jornvall, H., and Klein, G. (1980): Purification and biochemical characterization of the Epstein-Barr virus-determined nuclear antigen and an associated protein with a 53,000 dalton subunit. *J. Virol.*, 35:592–602.
26. Lusky, M., and Botchan, M. (1981): Inhibition of SV40 replication in simian cells by specific pBR 322 DNA sequences. *Nature*, 293:79–81.
27. Maltzman, W., Oren, M., and Levine, A. J. (1981): The structural relationships between 54000-molecular-weight cellular tumor antigens detected in viral- and non viral-transformed cells. *Virology*, 112:145–156.
28. May, E., Jeltsch, J. M., and Gannon, F. (1981): Characterization of a gene encoding a 115 K super-T antigen expressed by a SV40-transformed rat cell line. *Nucleic Acids Res.*, 9:4111–4128.
29. May, E., Kress, M., Daya-Grosjean, L., Monier, R., and May, P. (1981): Mapping of the viral mRNA encoding a super-T antigen of 115,000 daltons expressed in SV40-transformed rat cell lines. *J. Virol.*, 37:24–35.
30. May, E., Lasne, L., Prives, C., Bordé, J., and May, P. (1982): Study of the functional activities concomitantly retained by 115 K Super T antigen, an evolutionary variant of SV40 large T antigen expressed in transformed rat cells. *(To be submitted.)*
31. May, E., May, P., and Weil, R. (1971): Analysis of the events leading to SV40-induced chromosome replication and mitosis in primary mouse kidney cell cultures. *Proc. Natl. Acad. Sci. USA*, 68:1208–1211.
32. May, P., Kress, M., Lange, M., and May, E. (1980): New genetic information expressed in SV40-transformed cells: Characterization of the 55 K proteins and evidence for unusual SV40 mRNAs. *Cold Spring Harbor Symp. Quant. Biol.*, 44:189–200.
33. May, P., May, E., and Bordé, J. (1976): Stimulation of cellular RNA synthesis in mouse-kidney cell cultures infected with SV40 virus. *Exp. Cell. Res.*, 100:433–436.
34. Melero, J. A., Stitt, D. T., Mangel, W. F., and Carroll, R. B. (1979): Identification of new polypeptide species (48-55 K) immunoprecipitable by antiserum to purified large-T antigen and present in SV40-infected and transformed cells. *Virology*, 93:466–480.
35. Melero, J. A., Tur, S., and Carroll, R. B. (1980): Host nuclear proteins expressed in simian virus 40-transformed and -infected cells. *Proc. Natl. Acad. Sci. USA*, 77:97–101.
36. McCormick, F., Clark, R., Harlow, E., and Tjian, R. (1981): SV40 T antigen binds specifically to a cellular 53 K protein in vitro. *Nature*, 292:63–65.
37. McCormick, F., and Harlow, E. (1980): Association of a murine 53,000-dalton phosphoprotein with simian virus 40 large-T antigen in transformed cells. *J. Virol.*, 34:213–224.
38. McCutchan, J. H., and Pagano, J. S. (1968): Enhancement of the infectivity of simian virus 40 deoxyribonucleic acid with diethyl-aminoethyl-dextran. *J. Natl. Cancer Inst.*, 41:351–356.
39. Milner, J., and McCormick, F. (1980): Lymphocyte stimulation: Concanavalin A induces the expression of a 53 K protein. *Cell Biol. Int. Rep.*, 4:663–667.

40. Milner, J., and Milner, S. (1981): SV40-53 K antigen: A possible role for 53 K in normal cells. *Virology*, 112:785–788.
41. Mora, P. T., Chandrasekaran, K., and McFarland, V. W. (1980): An embryo protein induced by SV40 virus transformation of mouse cells. *Nature*, 288:722–724.
42. Oren, M., Maltzman, W., and Levine, A. J. (1981): Post-translational regulation of the 54 K cellular tumor antigen in normal and transformed cells. *Mol. Cell. Biol.*, 1:101–110.
43. Pintel, D., Bouck, N., and Di Mayorca, G. (1981): Separation of lytic and transforming functions of the simian virus 40 A region: Two mutants which are temperature sensitive for lytic functions have opposite effects on transformation. *J. Virol.*, 38:518–528.
44. Reddy, V. B., Thimmappaya, B., Dhar, R., Subramanian, K. N., Zain, B. S., Pan, J., Ghosh, P. K., Celma, M. L., and Weissman, S. M. (1978): The genome of simian virus 40. *Science*, 200:494–502.
45. Rotter, V., Boss, M. A., and Baltimore, D. (1981): Increased concentration of an apparently identical cellular protein in cells transformed by either Abelson murine leukemia virus or other transforming agents. *J. Virol.*, 38:336–346.
46. Simmons, D. T. (1980): Characterization of Tau antigens isolated from uninfected and simian virus 40-infected monkey cells and papovavirus-transformed cells. *J. Virol.*, 36:519–525.
47. Simmons, D. T., Martin, M. A., Mora, P. T., and Chang, C. (1980): Relationship among Tau antigens isolated from various lines of simian virus 40-transformed cells. *J. Virol.*, 34:650–657.
48. Smith, A. E., Smith, R., and Paucha, E. (1979): Characterization of different tumor antigens present in cells transformed by simian virus 40. *Cell*, 18:335–346.
49. Van der Eb, A. J., and Graham, F. L. (1980): Assay of transforming activity of tumor virus DNA. In: *Methods in Enzymology, Vol. 65. Nucleic Acids, Part 1*, edited by L. Grossman and K. Moldave, pp. 826–839. Academic Press, New York.

Advances in Viral Oncology, Volume 2, edited by
George Klein. Raven Press, New York © 1982.

The Mechanisms Regulating the Levels of the Cellular p53 Tumor Antigen in Transformed Cells

A. J. Levine, M. Oren, N. Reich, and P. Sarnow

*State University of New York at Stony Brook, Department of Microbiology,
School of Medicine, Stony Brook, New York 11794*

Many transformed cells in culture express high levels of a cellular phosphoprotein, termed p53 (4,5,18,22,35). In contrast, their non-transformed counterparts, such as Balb 3T3 or primary fibroblasts, contain between one-tenth to one-one hundredth the levels of p53 that are found in homologous transformed cell lines (4,23). p53 can be defined as a tumor antigen because animals bearing SV40-induced tumors (17,22) or hyperimmunized with a methylcholanthrene transformed cell line (5) produce anti p53 antibodies. These antibodies have been employed to detect and study the p53 cellular tumor antigen in normal and transformed cells. Cells transformed by a wide variety of agents express high levels of p53—chemical transformants such as meth A (5) or DMBA (25), irradiation leukemias (5), spontaneous transformants 3T12 (5,25), embryonal carcinoma cells derived from genetically predisposed mice (22,23), and cells transformed by RNA (5,35) and DNA viruses (4,18,22,24, 35,36). Although p53 was first described in the murine system (18,22), it has become clear that a homologous protein is regulated by or with the transformed state in human, monkey, hamster, and rat cells (4,13,22,40). Some monoclonal antibodies to the murine p53 protein cross-react with the homologous p53 proteins from all of these species (11,12), whereas other monoclonal antibodies are species- or primate-specific (48). In addition, the p53 proteins from human, monkey, mouse, and rat share some, but not all, methionine-containing tryptic peptides indicating a conservation of structure, and presumably function, over evolutionary time scales (40). The methionine-containing tryptic peptides of p53 proteins obtained from a variety of different murine-transformed cell lines are very similar to each other or identical (25). Thus, the levels of the p53 cellular tumor antigen are regulated either by or with the transformed state, independent of the agent involved in causing transformation and in a diverse number of species.

Because many transformed cell lines express high levels of p53 whereas normal cells have low levels of this protein, the mechanisms involved in regulating the level of this protein are of some interest. This chapter describes experiments that study this question, utilizing three different systems—SV40-transformed cells, adenovirus-transformed cells, and embryonal carcinoma cells. Surprisingly, p53 appears to be regulated differently in SV40-transformed cells and embryonal carcinoma cells. In SV40-transformed 3T3 cells and normal 3T3 cells, the levels of translatable p53 mRNA were found to be about the same (28) even though there were 10- to 100-fold higher amounts of p53 protein in the SV40-transformed cells. Apparently p53 is synthesized in both normal and transformed cells at about the same rate. However, the p53 protein in 3T3 cells is unstable and is degraded (or fails to react with antibody) rapidly with a half-life of about 20 to 60 min (28). The levels of p53 are higher in SV40-transformed cells because the p53 protein is not rapidly turned over, having a half-life of greater than 20 hr in these cells (28). The increased stability of the p53 protein in SV40-transformed cells may be a result of its physical association with the SV40 large T-antigen (6,18,22,26). In support of this idea is the observation that the SV40 large T-antigen is required to stimulate and maintain the high levels of p53 observed in SV40-infected and SV40-transformed cells (23).

The F9 embryonal carcinoma cell line has high levels of p53 when compared with normal cells (22) and produces tumors in syngeneic mice (10,39). When F9 cells are treated with retinoic acid and cAMP, they differentiate, predominantly into endoderm-like cells (43,44). After differentiation, the levels of p53 decline. The decline in the level of p53 on differentiation of F9 cells is accompanied by a decline in the level of translatable p53-specific mRNA, as determined by the ability to translate this mRNA in a reticulocyte system *in vitro* (29). The half-life of the p53 protein itself in F9 cells and differentiated cells is about the same (3 to 4 hr) in contrast to the 3T3-SV3T3 system. Clearly, the decline in p53 protein levels in benign differentiated cells is accompanied by a decline in translatable p53 mRNA.

It appears that there are at least two mechanisms involved in regulating the levels of p53 in normal and transformed cells: (a) posttranslational protein turnover in the 3T3-SV3T3 system and (b) transcriptional and/or translational control in the F9 embryonal carcinoma-differentiated cell system. Hence, two diverse transforming agents can act at different levels of regulation to achieve the same result—increased amounts of p53 in the transformed cell.

POSTTRANSLATIONAL REGULATION OF THE p53 CELLULAR ANTIGEN IN 3T3 AND SV40-TRANSFORMED 3T3 CELLS

Subconfluent cell cultures of secondary baby mouse fibroblasts, Balb 3T3 cells, and SV40-transformed Balb 3T3 cells (SVT2) were labeled with ^{35}S-methionine for 4 hr as described previously (22,28). The soluble proteins were extracted from these cells and these extracts were incubated with SV40 tumor serum to immunoprecipitate p53 and the SV40 T-antigen. In each case the same number of ^{35}S-methionine cpm were employed in the immunoprecipitation reaction and sufficient antibody was employed so as to be in antibody excess. These precipitations were analyzed by SDS-polyacrylamide gel electrophoresis. The gels were then exposed to X-ray film to obtain an autoradiogram indicating the levels of p53 proteins in the three different cell extracts. Several exposures of the autoradiogram were employed (8) to quantitate by densitometer tracings the level of p53 synthesized and present in the baby mouse fibroblasts, 3T3, and SV3T3 cell cultures (28). Table 1 presents the results of this com-

TABLE 1. *Comparison of the levels of p53 detected in baby mouse kidney fibroblasts, 3T3, or SV3T3 cell cultures* in vivo, *and synthesized by p53 mRNA* in vitro

Cell line	Relative levels of p53	
	p53-labeled *in vivo*	p53 translated *in vitro*
3T3	8.6 – 22.1	156 – 159
Mouse fibroblasts	5.7	48.3
SV3T3	100[a]	100[a]

[a]SV3T3 levels have been normalized to 100 units for comparison with other cell lines.

parison. The SV3T3 cell line contained 5- to 20-fold higher levels of p53 than either the secondary mouse fibroblasts or the 3T3 cells when these proteins were labeled for 4 hr with ^{35}S-methionine.

To examine the levels of p53 mRNA in these cell lines, cytoplasmic mRNA was obtained from these same cell cultures (28). This RNA was employed to prime an *in vitro* protein synthesis reaction using a rabbit reticulocyte system in the presence of ^{35}S-methionine. The levels of p53-specific mRNA were inferred from the levels of p53 protein synthesized *in vitro* and immunoprecipitated with SV40 tumor serum (28). Employing the mRNAs from 3T3 cells, baby mouse fibroblasts, and SV3T3 cells at concentrations optimal for *in vitro* translation, the levels of translatable mRNA from all three cell cultures were similar (Table 1). A comparison of the levels of p53 labeled in cell cultures *in vivo* or synthesized *in vitro* indicates that normal cells (3T3 and baby mouse fibroblasts) and transformed cells (SV3T3) contain roughly equal levels of p53-translatable mRNAs. In contrast, the levels of p53 protein labeled *in vivo* are 5- to 20-fold greater in SV3T3 cells than the normal cells in culture (Table 1).

Two lines of evidence indicate that *in vitro* translation of p53 is a fair reflection of the levels of p53-specific mRNA found in normal or transformed cells. First, the peptide maps of p53 synthesized in cell culture *in vivo* or *in vitro*, by the reticulocyte system, were very similar or identical (25,28). Second, the levels of p53 synthesized *in vitro* were proportional to the amounts of mRNA used to prime the reaction in both 3T3- and SV3T3-derived mRNA populations (Fig. 1). Thus it appears that the reticulocyte *in vitro* translation assay is a fair reflection of the levels of p53-specific translatable mRNA in a cell culture.

Several possible explanations exist for the unusual result that the levels of p53-translatable mRNAs are about the same in normal and transformed cells, but the level of p53 proteins detected by *in vivo* labeling of cells in culture are 5- to 20-fold greater in transformed

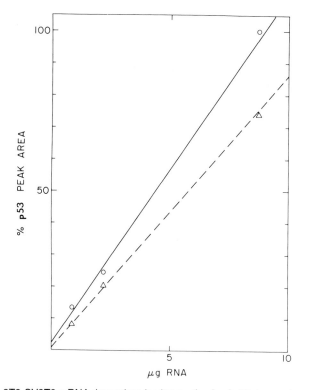

FIG. 1. 3T3-SV3T3 mRNA dependent *in vitro* synthesis of p53. Increasing amounts of cytoplasmic RNA from either 3T3 *(triangle)* or SVT2 *(circle)* cells were translated in the reticulocyte lysate system and immunoprecipitated with anti p53 serum. Total samples were run on a polyacrylamide gel and the amount of p53 made *in vitro* was determined by densitometer tracing of the resultant autoradiogram. The values of p53 are presented as percentage of the highest value observed in this experiment.

cells than in normal cells. For example, 3T3 cells and SV3T3 cells might synthesize equal amounts of p53, but this protein could be rapidly degraded in 3T3 cells. SV3T3 cells, on the other hand, would contain a more stable form of p53, possibly due to the fact that this cellular protein is physically complexed with SV40 large T-antigen (6,18,22,26). To test this idea, a pulse chase experiment was performed. 3T3 cells and SV3T3 cells were labeled with ^{35}S-methionine for 2 hr after which the medium was removed and the cultures were refed with medium not containing the radioisotope (28). At several times during this chase period, cell cultures were harvested and the levels of p53 protein were measured as described previously. Figure 2 presents the autoradiogram showing the levels of p53 synthesized in 3T3 and SV3T3 cells during the pulse labeling time (0 time of the chase) and the levels of p53 retained in the cells after a chase period of 3, 10, or 22 hr. The chase of the radioisotope was effective, as the total incorporation of ^{35}S-methionine into TCA-precipitable proteins did not increase during this chase period. In SV3T3 cells, both the SV40 T-antigen and p53 were stable over the 22 hr-chase period. In 3T3 cells, p53 was detectable after the 2-hr labeling period (Fig. 2: 3T3, 0 hr), but by a 3-hr chase period little or no p53 was observed by immunoprecipitation using anti p53 antibodies. Thus, p53 appears to be rapidly turned over in 3T3 cells. Based on several experiments, the half-life of p53 in 3T3 cells was determined to be 20 to 60 min whereas the half-life of this same protein in SV3T3 cells was greater than 20 hr. Since antibody is the exclusive tool employed to detect p53 in all these experiments, it remains possible that p53 in 3T3 cells is not necessarily degraded rapidly. The p53 protein could take on an altered conformation or form that is no longer accessible to detection by the antibody, or it could become an insoluble protein not extracted into the soluble antigen pool and detected by immunoprecipitation.

In any case, it is clear that the high levels of p53 in SV40-transformed cells are due to the accumulation of a stable soluble protein. The levels of translatable p53 mRNA in 3T3 and SV3T3 cell lines are roughly equivalent (Table 1, Fig. 1); it is therefore

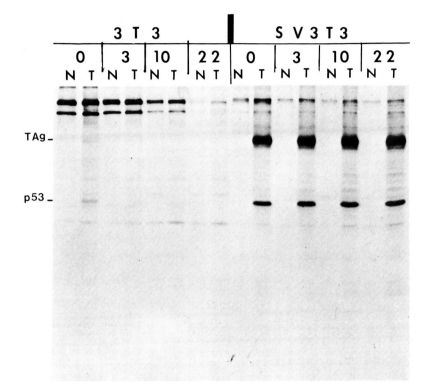

FIG. 2. Pulse chase analysis of p53 *in vivo* in 3T3 and SV3T3 cells. Cells were pulse labeled for 2 hr with (^{35}S) methionine. The cells were then exhaustively washed with methionine-containing medium and incubated in this media for the indicated chase periods (hr). Proteins were extracted and equal amounts of trichloroacetic acid insoluble radioactivity were immunoprecipitated with anti p53 serum and analyzed. The autoradiogram of the 3T3 cells was exposed for 5 days and that of the SV3T3 cells was exposed for 2 days (2).

likely that the protein itself is synthesized at comparable rates in both cell lines. In 3T3 cells, p53 is either rapidly degraded after synthesis or assumes an altered form, not detectable by the normal assay procedures. The level of regulation of p53 in 3T3-SV3T3 cells thus appears to be at a posttranslational step, i.e., protein turnover or alteration. The possibility that translational control may contribute an additional effect has not been excluded.

TRANSCRIPTIONAL OR TRANSLATIONAL REGULATION OF THE p53 CELLULAR ANTIGEN IN EMBRYONAL CARCINOMAL CELLS UNDERGOING DIFFERENTIATION

Teratocarcinomas are tumors of pluripotent blastomeres derived from primordial germ cells (30,41,42). The tumors are composed of a malignant stem cell, called embryonal carcinoma cells (EC cells), and benign differentiated cells or tissue types derived from these EC cells (15,16,27,30,32,39,41,42). F9 cells (1) are an embryonal carcinoma cell line that normally does not differentiate in cell culture but, when exposed to retinoic acid and cAMP, will produce endoderm as the predominant cell type (43,44). EC cell lines, like F9 cells, contain high levels of p53 (22,23). A study was performed to follow the levels of p53 during differentiation of tumorigenic F9 cells into benign differentiated cells.

Cell cultures of F9 cells and F9 cells treated with retinoic acid and cAMP (44) for 4 days were labeled with ^{35}S-methionine for 4 hr. The soluble proteins were extracted and p53 levels were determined by immunoprecipitation as described previously. Figure 3 presents the autoradiograms from this experiment. The levels of p53 protein decrease about fivefold after differentiation of F9 cells. This decline in p53 levels found in differentiated cells is probably an underestimate because about 5% of these cells in the retinoic acid-treated culture remained F9 EC cells with high levels of p53. Infection of the differentiated cells with SV40 restores the high levels of p53 observed in these cells (Fig. 3). Thus, differentiation of tumorigenic embryonal carcinoma cells into a benign cell type results in a decrease in the levels of p53.

To determine if the half-life of the p53 protein is shorter in differentiated cells than in F9 EC cells, a pulse chase experiment was carried out in these two cultures. F9 cells and differentiated cells were labeled with ^{35}S-methionine for an hour followed by a 10-hr chase period in unlabeled medium. Figure 4 presents the autoradiogram of the SDS-polyacrylamide gel, showing the levels

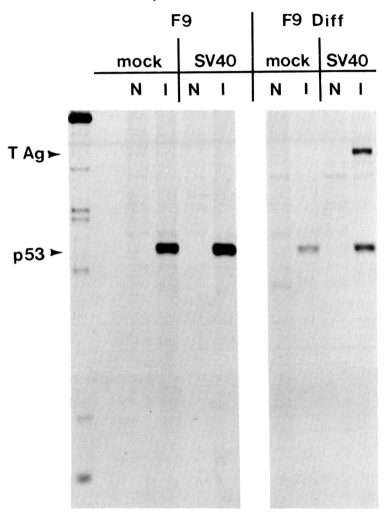

FIG. 3. Levels of p53 in F9 cells and differentiated F9 cells. F9 cells were differentiated in the presence of 10^{-7} M retinoic acid and 10^{-3} M dibutyryl cAMP for 4 days. The F9 cells and the differentiated cells were either infected with SV40 virus or mock infected. At 16 hr postinfection, cultures were labeled with (^{35}S) methionine for 3 hr. Proteins were extracted and equal amounts of trichloroacetic acid insoluble radioactivity were immunoprecipitated and analyzed on polyacrylamide gels. Left lane displays adenovirus type 5 marker proteins.

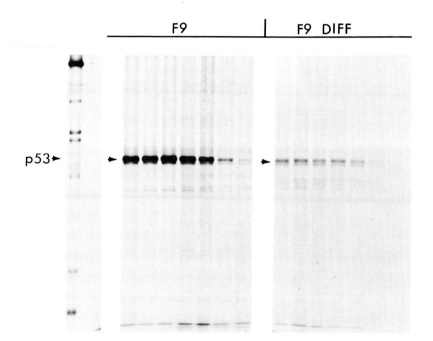

FIG. 4. Pulse-chase analysis of p53 *in vitro* in F9 and differentiated cells. F9 cells and their differentiated counterparts (refer to Fig. 3) were pulse labeled with (³⁵S)-methionine for 1 hr. The cells were then exhaustively washed in methionine-containing medium and incubated in this medium for 0, 0.45, 1.5, 2.5, 3.5, 6, or 10 hr. Proteins were extracted, immunoprecipitated with anti-p53 serum, and analyzed on a poly-acrylamide gel.

of p53 in F9 and differentiated cell cultures, detected by immuno-precipitation with p53 antibodies. From this experiment it is clear that the levels (at all times) of p53 are lower (about fivefold) in the differentiated cells than in the F9 EC cells. The half-lives of p53 in F9 cells and the differentiated cells were about the same, i.e., approximately 3.5 hr, indicating that protein turnover was not a major factor in regulating p53 levels in F9 cells or their differentiated counterpart.

To examine the p53 mRNA levels in F9 and the differentiated cells, the following experiment was carried out. Cytoplasmic mRNA from F9 cells and the differentiated cells was obtained and translated *in vitro* in a reticulocyte system (29). Again the analysis of the levels of mRNA were quantitated by the levels of p53 synthesized *in vitro* and detected with anti p53 antibody (Table 2). Figure 5 presents a dose response curve with increasing levels of mRNA priming the

TABLE 2. *Comparison of the levels of p53 detected in untreated and retinoic acid treated F9 cells* in vivo, *and synthesized by p53 mRNA* in vitro

	Relative levels of p53	
Cells	p53 labeled *in vivo*	p53 translated *in vitro*
F9	100.0	100.0
F9, Retinoic acid treated	24.1	16.3

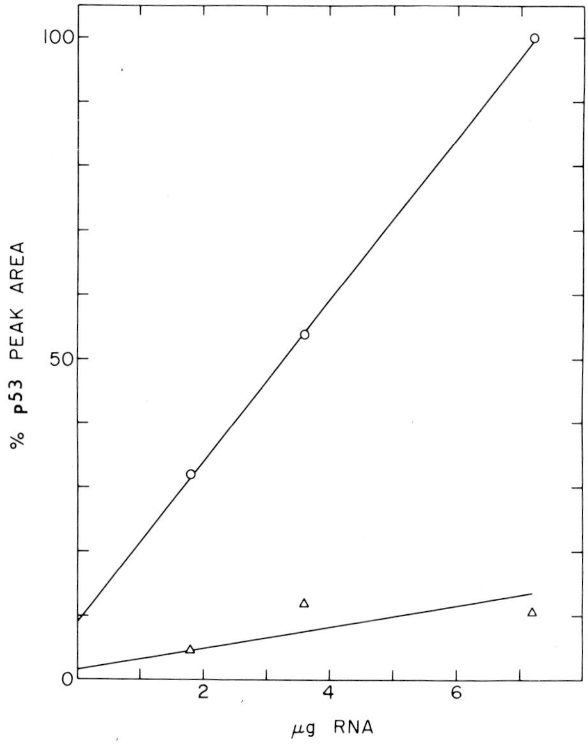

FIG. 5. F9-differentiated mRNA-dependent *in vitro* synthesis of p53. Experimental details are essentially as described in the legend to Fig. 1. *Circle*, untreated cells; *triangle*, retinoic acid- and cAMP-treated F9 cells.

in vitro translation reaction. From these data it is clear that F9 cells contain sixfold higher levels of translatable p53 mRNA than was detectable in the differentiated cell culture. In the case of F9 cells differentiating into a benign cell type, the level of p53 does not appear to be regulated at a posttranslational step like SV40-transformed cells. The difference in levels of translatable p53 mRNA in the F9 differentiation system indicates a control mechanism at the level of gene transcription, although it remains possible that translational control could also account for these results.

THE ADENOVIRUS E1b-58K TUMOR ANTIGEN IS PHYSICALLY ASSOCIATED WITH p53 IN ADENOVIRUS-TRANSFORMED MOUSE CELLS

Like SV40-transformed mouse cells (18,22), adenovirus-transformed mouse cells (Ho and Williams, *personal communication*) express high levels of p53. To investigate the possibility that an adenovirus-encoded tumor antigen, like the SV40 large T-antigen, was physically associated with p53 in these cells, the following experiment was performed. Three different cell cultures—adenovirus-infected HeLa cells, SV40-transformed mouse cells (SVT2), and adenovirus-transformed mouse cells (Ho and Williams, *unpublished data*) (C3H-DC3)—were labeled with ^{35}S-methionine for a 4-hr period. The soluble proteins were then extracted from these cells and the extracts incubated with either antibodies from hamsters bearing adenovirus-induced tumors (Ad2, tumor serum), a monoclonal antibody to p53 (α53) (3), or normal serum. The immunoprecipitates from these reactions were analyzed as usual, and the autoradiogram that resulted from this experiment is presented in Fig. 6. In adenovirus-infected HeLa cells, the Ad2 tumor serum detected the E1b-58K viral tumor antigen (8,20,21,33,34,36,37). The αp53 monoclonal antibody and the normal serum did not detect any proteins. HeLa cells do not express detectable levels of p53 (4,36). In the SV40-transformed cell extract, the αp53 monoclonal antibody immunoprecipitated p53 and its associated SV40 large T-antigen (18,22). The Ad2 serum and normal serum did not detect any pro-

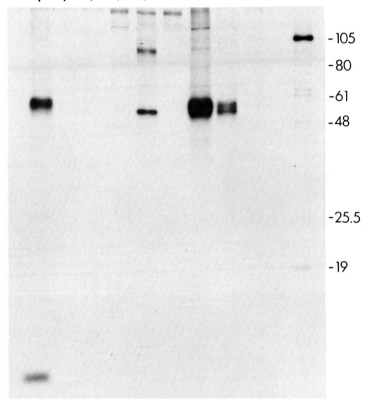

FIG. 6. Immunoprecipitation of adenovirus (Elb-58K), SV40 (T-antigen), and associated cellular proteins (p53) from adenovirus-infected, SV40-transformed, and adenovirus-transformed cells. HeLa cells were infected with adenovirus type 5 (100 pfu/cell) and labeled with ^{35}S-methionine at 12 to 16 hr postinfection. SV40-transformed 3T3 cells (SVT2) and adenovirus-transformed C3H mouse kidney cells (C3H-DC3) were labeled for 4 hr with the same isotope. Soluble cell extracts were prepared and immunoprecipitated (33): Ad2-serum *(Ad2)* was obtained from a hamster bearing an adenovirus induced tumor (33); $\alpha p53$ is a monoclonal antibody to the cellular p53 protein (3); *ns* is normal hamster serum. The immunoprecipitates were analyzed by SDS-polyacrylamide gel electrophoresis and the autoradiogram is presented.

teins. In the adenovirus-transformed mouse cell culture (C3H-DC3), the Ad2 tumor serum immunoprecipitated the Elb-58K viral tumor antigen and a second associated protein giving rise to a doublet or broader band at the 53 to 58,000 MW range. The αp53 monoclonal antibody immunoprecipitated p53 and coimmunoprecipitated a second protein, the Elb-58K adenovirus tumor antigen. Based on these results, the following is clear: (a) the Ad2 tumor serum does not cross-react with p53 (see SVT2 lanes), (b) the p53 monoclonal antibody does not cross-react with the adenovirus Elb-58K protein (see Ad5-HeLa lanes), and (c) since the Ad2 tumor serum and the p53 monoclonal antibodies detect both these proteins in the adenovirus-transformed mouse cells, the Elb-58K adenovirus tumor antigen and the p53 antigen must be in a physical association in the transformed cell extract.

This experiment demonstrates that the SV40 large T-antigen and the adenovirus Elb-58K tumor antigen are found in a physical complex with this murine cellular protein p53 in transformed cells. The evidence that the same cellular protein is physically complexed with these two viral tumor antigens (Fig. 6) rests on a shared antigen determinant detected by the αp53 monoclonal antibody. To demonstrate that the p53 protein associated with the SV40 and adenovirus tumor antigens was indeed the same cellular protein, a comparison of the peptides from these two proteins was undertaken. The p53 protein from SV40-transformed cells was coimmunoprecipitated with a monoclonal antibody directed against the SV40 large T-antigen and the associated p53 protein isolated from an SDS-polyacrylamide gel slice. The p53 from the adenovirus-transformed cell line (C3H-DC3) was coimmunoprecipitated with Ad2 tumor serum, which only detects the Elb-58K protein (see Fig. 6), and the associated p53 was isolated from an SDS-polyacrylamide gel slice. The ^{35}S-methionine-labeled p53 proteins from SV40- and adenovirus-transformed mouse cells were treated with the *Staphylococcus aureus* V8 protease and the partial peptide cleavages were compared in an SDS-polyacrylamide gel (2). Figure 7 presents the results of these peptide map comparisons. From these data it is clear that the p53 proteins associated with the SV40 T-antigen and the adenovirus Elb-

C3H-DC3-p53   SVT2-p53

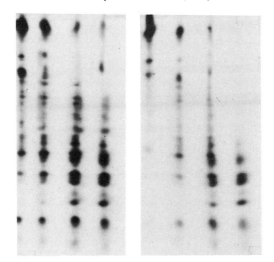

FIG. 7. Limited proteolysis peptide map of the cellular p53 protein from adenovirus-transformed cells (C3H-DC3-p53) and SV40-transformed cells (SVT2-p53). ^{35}S-methionine-labeled cell extracts were prepared and the Elb-58K antigen was immunoprecipitated by the polyclonal serum Ad2 (specific for the Elb-58K protein only), while the SV40 T-antigen was immunoprecipitated by a monoclonal antibody to T-antigen (11). The coimmunoprecipitated p53 cellular proteins were cut out of the gel and a limited proteolysis peptide map (2) was obtained by treating the protein with increasing concentrations of *S. aureus* V8 protease *(left to right)*. An autoradiogram of the SDS-polyacrylamide gel is shown.

58K T-antigen are very similar or identical. Thus, the same cellular protein, p53, is physically associated with two different viral tumor antigens—the SV40 large T-antigen and the adenovirus Elb-58K tumor antigen—in different virus-transformed cells.

DISCUSSION AND SPECULATIONS ON THE FUNCTION OF THE p53 TUMOR ANTIGEN

The SV40 large tumor antigen and the adenovirus Elb-58K tumor antigen each form large molecular weight, multimeric complexes with the same cellular protein, p53 (26,36). If it is assumed that these complexes have a functional significance, the p53 should have an effect on the function of the SV40 large T-antigen and the adenovirus Elb-58K gene product (and/or vice versa). Genetic analyses with the SV40 and adenovirus tumor antigens have elucidated several functions of these two viral proteins. Both the SV40 large T-antigen (47) and the adenovirus Elb protein(s) (7) are required for transformation of cells in culture by these viruses. The SV40 large T-antigen is required to initiate each round of viral DNA replication (45) and is involved in the stimulation of cellular DNA synthesis after virus infection (9,49). Similarly, the adenovirus Elb gene product(s) is required for viral DNA synthesis in, as yet, an undetermined fashion (14,34). The SV40 large T-antigen can modulate down early viral transcripts (47) and modulate up some cellular transcripts (T. Schutzbank et al., *unpublished data*). The SV40 T-antigen can also regulate the levels of a variety of cellular enzyme activities (thymidine kinase, deoxycytidine kinase) that normally are controlled by or with the growth rate of a cell culture (31). Thus, the SV40 large T-antigen can modulate the levels of viral and cellular gene products. Similarly, the Elb gene product(s) can modulate the levels of several adenovirus gene products (adenovirus E2 and E3 gene products) (14,34). It is clear from this analysis that the SV40 large T-antigen and the adenovirus Elb-58K protein may share a number of functional properties in addition to their interaction with the same cellular protein, p53.

Since transformed cells express higher levels of p53 than normal cells (4,5,18,22,35,36) and transformed cells replicate under conditions where normal cells usually do not grow, it is assumed that p53 acts in a positive fashion to direct or alter the function of these SV40 and adenovirus tumor antigens. The interactions between p53 and the SV40 T-antigen and adenovirus Elb-58K protein could result in a chemical modification of the tumor antigens allowing them to function in some new manner. Alternatively, the oligomeric form of these viral-cellular protein complexes could function differently than the monomeric form of these proteins.

Since both the SV40 T-antigen and the adenovirus Elb-58K protein are involved in DNA replication and can alter viral and/or cellular gene expression, it is reasonable to assume that these viral proteins do so via interactions with several cellular proteins, and p53 is one such protein. In normal cells, p53 would be one of a complex of proteins involved in normal cellular DNA replication and/or the regulation of cellular genes that are enhanced during active growth. A close spacial relationship between origins of DNA replication and promoters for active gene transcription has already been proposed (38). The viral tumor antigens may well replace normal cellular proteins in these replication or gene regulation protein complexes. In this case, the viral proteins, SV40 T-antigen or Elb-58K protein, have evolved so as to interact with the cellular proteins in a DNA replication or transcriptional complex, better than the cellular protein that they replace. In this way a viral protein can usurp and take control of the DNA replication or the gene regulation complex utilizing it for viral replication or, in the case of a transformed cell, resulting in uncontrolled growth and a gene expression compatible with cell replication.

In the case of 3T3 cells, p53 is synthesized. It then functions, and the protein is degraded or turned over, keeping the levels of p53 in the cell low. This is a reflection of the normal cellular growth control, where replication and gene regulation protein complexes are at low levels and under control. By virtue of the fact that SV40 T-antigen enters the gene regulation and/or DNA replication protein complexes, these associations of proteins are stabilized and accumulate in the cell. Thus, SV40 T-antigen, which is required for cellular transformation (46) and is required to stimulate and maintain high levels of p53 in the transformed cell (23), stabilizes the p53 protein by virtue of forming a multimeric complex and increases the half-life of the protein in the cell. The higher levels of DNA replication and/or gene regulation complexes (a reflection of which is the higher levels of p53 in such cells) act in a positive fashion to keep on the cell growth phenotype called transformation. Some viruses, like SV40 and adenovirus, therefore, transform cells by providing a viral protein or tumor antigen that is more efficient at forming and stabilizing DNA replication and gene regulation protein complexes. These viral proteins have evolved so as to replace cellular functions and efficiently redirect the cellular regulatory mechanisms to the advantage of virus replication. In so doing, a by-product of this evolutionary strategy is the alteration of the cellular functions resulting in transformation.

This explanation of SV40 and adenovirus transformation now can be employed to understand cellular transformation by agents other than viruses. Alterations or mutations in a variety of cellular genes (e.g., by carcinogens or irradiation) could result, via chemical modification of proteins or enhanced levels of several proteins, in a stabilization of these DNA replication or gene regulation protein complexes. The constitutive synthesis and/or high stability of these gene regulation complexes (reflected by high p53 levels in any transformed cell) results in the transformed phenotype. In the case of F9 embryonal carcinoma cells, the transforming event results in a more stable p53-cellular protein complex (half-life of p53 in F9 cells is 3 to 4 hr, whereas in 3T3 cells the half-life of p53 is 20 to 60 min). After differentiation of F9 cells, the levels of p53 decline because transcriptional controls modulate down the expression of p53 to alter gene regulation and produce an endoderm cell type. The lower levels of p53 thus synthesized (and presumably other proteins in the DNA replication, gene regulation, protein complexes) result in a reversal of the transformed phenotype, producing a benign differentiated cell type with reduced p53 levels. In this case, part of the program involved in differentiation is to modulate down transcripts of genes whose protein products are involved in cellular replication complexes.

This hypothesis predicts that the normal function of p53 is to be involved in protein-protein interactions that result in either DNA replication (initiation of DNA replication) and/or the regulation of cellular genes (in a positive fashion) that must be actively expressed (transcribed) during cell growth or division. p53 might act transiently to modify chemically such positive regulators of DNA replication or transcription (like SV40 or adenovirus T-antigens or their presumed cellular equivalent) or it could form a stable complex with cellular or viral proteins to provide the positive regulation. A clear prediction of this hypothesis is a central role for p53 in the initiation of DNA replication and/or transcriptional initiation complexes for cellular genes (like thymidine kinase) regulated by or with the growth of the cell. The central role of SV40 T-antigen in DNA replication and its positive regulation of cellular genes involved in growth control (31,46), along with the formation of multimeric protein complexes between T-antigen and p53, is consistent with this prediction. The hypothetical cellular equivalent of SV40 T-antigen could thus be one target for chemical carcinogens and the resultant transformation event that they cause. Finally, the existence of cellular T-antigen analog, and its resultant p53-cellular T protein complex in actively growing cells, is yet another prediction of this model. The test of many of these ideas will have to await a more sophisticated experimental ability to initiate DNA synthesis *in vitro* or provide a positive control of transcriptional initiation events with specific cellular genes. Clearly, advances in basic questions of gene regulation go hand and hand with understanding the molecular basis of cellular transformation.

ACKNOWLEDGMENTS

The authors thank A. K. Teresky, P. K. Lundy, and C. Sullivan for technical assistance. We also thank Y. S. Ho and J. Williams for adenovirus-transformed mouse cell lines. This research was supported by grants CA28106, CA23033, CA28127, CA28146, and CA25166 from the National Cancer Institute to A. J. Levine.

REFERENCES

1. Bernstine, E. G., Hooper, M. L., Grandchamp, S., and Ephrussi, B. (1973): Alkaline phosphatase activity in mouse teratoma. *Proc. Natl. Acad. Sci. USA*, 70:3899–3903.
2. Cleveland, D., Fisher, S., Kirshner, M., and Laemmli, U. (1977): Peptide mapping by limited proteolysis in sodium dodecyl sulfate and analysis by gel electrophoresis. *J. Biol. Chem.*, 252:1102–1106.
3. Coffman, R. L., and Weissman, I. L. (1981): A monoclonal antibody that recognizes B cells and B cell precursors in mice. *J. Exp. Med.*, 153:269–279.
4. Crawford, L. V., Pim, D. C., Gurney, E. G., Goodfellow, P., and Taylor-Papadimitriou, J. (1981): Detection of a common feature in several human tumor cell lines: A 53,000-dalton protein. *Proc. Natl. Acad. Sci. USA*, 78:41–45.

5. DeLeo, A. B., Jay, G., Appella, E., Dubois, G. C., Law, L. W., and Old, L. J. (1979): Detection of a transformation-related antigen in chemically induced sarcomas and other transformed cells of the mouse. *Proc. Natl. Acad. Sci. USA*, 76:2420–2424.

6. Fanning, E., Nowak, B., and Burger, C. (1981): Detection and characterization of multiple forms of simian virus 40 large T-antigen. *J. Virol.*, 37:92–102.

7. Gallimore, P. H., Sharp, P. A., and Sambrook, J. (1974): Viral DNA in transformed cells: II. A study of the sequences of adenovirus 2 DNA in nine lines of transformed rat cells using specific fragments of the viral genome. *J. Mol. Biol.*, 89:49–72.

8. Gilead, Z., Jeng, Y. H., Wold, W. S. M., Sugawara, K., Rho, H. W., Harter, M. L., and Green, M. (1976): Immunological identification of two adenovirus induced early proteins possibly involved in cell transformation. *Nature*, 264:263–266.

9. Graessman, A., Graessman, M., and Muller, C. (1979): Simian virus 40 and polyoma virus gene expression explored by microinjection technique. In: *Current Topics in Microbiology and Immunology*, edited by W. Henle, H. Koprowski, and P. K. Vogt, Vol. 87, pp. 1–20. Springer-Verlag, New York.

10. Graham, C. F. (1977): Teratocarcinoma cells and normal mouse embryogenesis. In: *Concepts in Mammalian Embryogenesis*, edited by M. I. Sherman, pp. 315–394. MIT Press, Cambridge.

11. Gurney, E. G., Harrison, R. O., and Fenno, J. (1980): Monoclonal antibodies against simian virus 40 T antigens: Evidence for distinct subclasses of large T antigen and for similarities among nonviral T antigens. *J. Virol.*, 34:752–763.

12. Harlow, E., Crawford, L. V., Pim, D. C., and Williamson, N. (1981): Monoclonal antibodies specific for simian virus 40 tumor antigens. *J. Virol.*, 39:861–869.

13. Harlow, E., Pim, D. C., and Crawford, L. V. (1981): Complex of simian virus 40 large T antigen and host 53,000 molecular weight protein in monkey cells. *J. Virol.*, 37:564–573.

14. Jones, N., and Shenk, T. (1979): An adenovirus type 5 early gene function regulates expression of other early viral genes. *Proc. Natl. Acad. Sci. USA*, 76:3665–3669.

15. Kahn, B. W., and Ephrussi, B. (1970): Developmental potentialities of clonal *in vitro* cultures of mouse testicular teratomas. *J. Natl. Cancer Inst.*, 44:1015–1023.

16. Kleinsmith, L. J., and Pierce, Jr., G. B. (1964): Multipotentiality of single embryonal carcinoma cells. *Cancer Res.*, 24:1544–1552.

17. Kress, M., May, E., Cassingena, R., and May, P. (1979): Simian virus 40-transformed cells express new species of proteins precipitable by anti-simian virus tumor serum. *J. Virol.*, 31:472–483.

18. Lane, D. P., and Crawford, L. V. (1979): T antigen is bound to a host protein in SV40-transformed cells. *Nature*, 278:261–263.

19. Laskey, R. A., and Mills, A. D. (1975): Quantitative film detection of ³H and ¹⁴C in polyacrylamide gels by fluorography. *Eur. J. Biochem.*, 53:335–341.
20. Levinson, A. D., and Levine, A. J. (1977): The isolation and identification of the adenovirus group C tumor antigens. *Virology*, 76:1–11.
21. Levinson, A. D., and Levine, A. J. (1977): The group C adenovirus tumor antigens: Infected and transformed cells and a peptide map analysis. *Cell*, 11:871–879.
22. Linzer, D. I. H., and Levine, A. J. (1979): Characterization of a 54K dalton cellular SV40 tumor antigen present in SV40-transformed cells and uninfected embryonal carcinoma cells. *Cell*, 17:43–52.
23. Linzer, D. I. H., Maltzman, W., and Levine, A. J. (1979): The SV40: A gene product is required for the production of a 54,000 MW cellular tumor antigen. *Virology*, 98:308–318.
24. Luka, J., Jornvall, H., and Klein, G. (1980): Purification and biochemical characterization of the Epstein-Barr virus—determined nuclear antigen and an associated protein with a 53,000 dalton subunit. *J. Virol.*, 35:592–602.
25. Maltzman, W., Oren, M., and Levine, A. J. (1981): The structural relationships between 54,000 molecular weight cellular tumor antigens detected in viral and nonviral transformed cells. *Virology*, 112:145–156.
26. McCormick, F., and Harlow, E. (1980): Association of a murine 53,000 dalton phosphoprotein with simian virus 40 large T-antigen in transformed cells. *J. Virol.*, 34:213–224.
27. Mintz, B., and Illmensee, K. (1975): Normal genetically mosaic mice produced from malignant teratocarcinoma cells. *Proc. Natl. Acad. Sci. USA*, 72:3585–3589.
28. Oren, M., Maltzman, W., and Levine, A. J. (1981): Post-translational regulation of the 54K cellular tumor antigen in normal and transformed cells. *Mol. Cell. Biol.*, 1:101–110.
29. Oren, M., Reich, N., and Levine, A. J. (1982): The regulation of the cellular p53 tumor antigen in teratocarcinoma cells and their differentiated progeny, molecular and cellular biology. *(in press).*
30. Pierce, G. B. (1975): Teratocarcinoma: Introduction and perspectives. In: *Teratomas and Differentiation*, edited by M. I. Sherman and D. Solter, pp. 3–12. Academic Press, New York.
31. Postel, E. H., and Levine, A. J. (1976): The requirement of simian virus 40 gene A product for the stimulation of cellular thymidine kinase activity after viral infection. *Virology*, 73:206–215.
32. Rosenthal, M. D., Wishnow, R. M., and Sato, G. H. (1970): *In vitro* growth and differentiation of clonal populations of multipotential mouse cells derived from 2 transplantable testicular teratocarcinomas. *J. Natl. Cancer Inst.*, 44:1001–1009.
33. Ross, S. R., Flint, S. J., and Levine, A. J. (1980): Identification of the adenovirus early proteins and their genomic map positions. *Virology*, 100:419–432.

34. Ross, S. R., Levine, A. J., Galos, R. S., Williams, J., and Shenk, T. (1980): Early viral proteins in HeLa cells infected with adenovirus type 5 host range mutants. *Virology*, 103:475–492.
35. Rotter, V., Boss, M. A., and Baltimore, D. (1981): Increased concentrations of an apparently identical cellular protein in cells transformed by either abelson murine leukemia virus or other transforming agents. *J. Virol.*, 38:336–346.
36. Sarnow, P., Ho, Y., Williams, J., and Levine, A. J. (1982): The adenovirus Elb-58K tumor antigen and SV40 large tumor antigen are physically associated with the same 54K cellular protein. *Cell, (in press)*.
37. Schrier, P. I., van der Elsen, P. J., Hertoghs, J. J. L., and van der Eb, A. J. (1979): Characterization of tumor antigens in cells transformed by fragments of adenovirus type 5 DNA. *Virology*, 99:372–385.
38. Seidman, M. M., Levine, A. J., and Weintraub, H. (1979): The asymmetric segregation of parental nucleosomes during chromosome replication. *Cell*, 18:439–449.
39. Sherman, M. I., Matthaei, K. I., and Schindler, J. (1981): Studies on the mechanism of induction of embryonal carcinoma cell differentiation by retinoic acid. *Ann. N.Y. Acad. Sci.*, 359:192–199.
40. Simmons, D. T., Martin, M. A., Mora, P. T., and Chang, C. (1980): Relationship among tau antigens isolated from various lines of simian virus 40 transformed cells. *J. Virol.*, 34:650–657.
41. Solter, D., and Damjanov, I. (1979): Teratocarcinoma and the expression of oncodevelopmental genes. *Methods Cancer Res.*, 18:277–332.
42. Stevens, L. C. (1967): The biology of teratomas. In: *Advances in Morphogenesis*, edited by M. Abercrombie and J. Brachet, pp. 1–31. Academic Press, New York.
43. Strickland, S., and Mahdavi, V. (1978): The induction of differentiation in teratocarcinoma stem cells by retinoic acid. *Cell*, 15:393–403.
44. Strickland, S., Smith, K. E., and Marotti, K. R. (1980): Hormonal induction of differentiation in teratocarcinoma stem cells: Generation of parietal endoderm by retinoic acid and dibutyryl cAMP. *Cell*, 21:347–355.
45. Tegtmeyer, P. (1972): Simian virus 40 deoxyribonucleic acid synthesis: The viral replicon. *J. Virol.*, 10:591–598.
46. Tegtmeyer, P. (1975): Function of simian virus 40 gene A in transforming infection. *J. Virol.*, 15:613–618.
47. Tegtmeyer, P., Schwartz, M., Collins, J. K., and Rundell, K. (1975): Regulation of tumor antigen synthesis by simian virus 40 gene A. *J. Virol.*, 16:168–178.
48. Thomas, R., Sullivan, C., and Levine, A. J. (1982): Primate-specific p53 monoclonal antibodies. *(in preparation)*.
49. Tjian, R., Fey, G., and Graessman, A. (1978): Biological activity of purified simian virus 40 T antigen proteins. *Proc. Natl. Acad. Sci. USA*, 75:1279–1283.

Advances in Viral Oncology, Volume 2, edited by
George Klein. Raven Press, New York © 1982.

Host Nuclear Phosphoproteins That Complex Simian Virus 40 Large T Antigen

Robert B. Carroll, Andrea S. Blum, and
Daniel S. Greenspan

*Department of Pathology, New York University Medical School,
New York, New York 10016*

A new class of nuclear, host-encoded phosphoproteins (Mr = 48 to 55K) has been found tightly and specifically complexed with simian virus 40 (SV40) large T antigen (T Ag) in extracts of all cells thus far examined, after infection or transformation by the virus. The expression of the host protein(s) is readily detectable only in the presence of a functional A locus, which encodes T antigen, suggesting the host protein is one of the targets of T Ag, and may modulate one of the biological activities of T Ag. T Ag is necessary for both (a) viral replication in permissive monkey cells, in which case it both induces the host replicative enzymes (46) and initiates each round of DNA synthesis (40), and (b) apparently for oncogenic transformation (1,25,46). It is not clear in which or how many of the biological activities of the viral T Ag the host protein participates. However, most significantly, the same protein(s) has been detected at high levels, in the absence of T Ag, in cells transformed by a number of other carcinogenic agents (chemicals, various RNA and DNA tumor viruses, radiation) and in tumors of both animals and humans, as is outlined by a number of the authors of this volume. This strongly suggests that (a) there is host coding of the protein, (b) the host protein is involved in the transforming activity of T Ag, and (c) it participates in a mechanism of transformation common to a number of carcinogens.

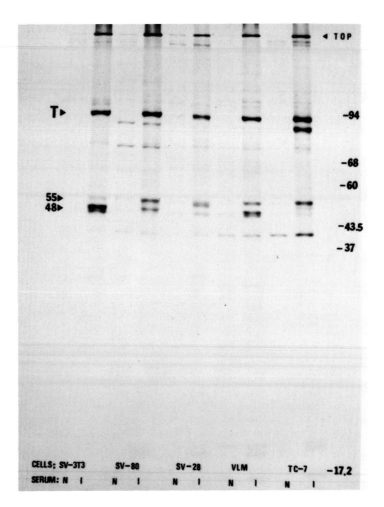

FIG. 1. Survey of immunoprecipitable polypeptides from SV40-transformed and -infected cells using antitumor serum. **Left:** Cells were labeled with [^{35}S]methionine for 20 to 22 hr. TC7 cells were infected with wild-type SV40 at moi = 5 and labeled with [^{35}S]methionine from 30 to 48 hr postinfection. Immunoprecipitation and electrophoresis were done as previously described (2). *N* denotes normal hamster serum and *I* denotes antitumor hamster serum. The numbers at the right correspond to the positions of molecular-weight markers, expressed in thousands. (From ref. 28, with permission.) **Right:** Cells were labeled with 70 μCi/ml of [^{32}P]orthophosphate in DMEM 10% calf serum and processed as indicated at left. T indicates large T Ag and 55 and 48 indicate the positions of the corresponding proteins, expressed in thousands.

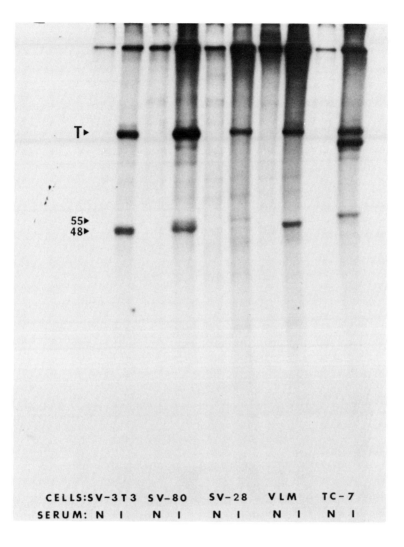

CELLS: SV-3T3   SV-80   SV-28   VLM   TC-7
SERUM: N I   N I   N I   N I   N I

The purpose of this chapter is to present our work characterizing the host nuclear phosphoprotein, with particular emphasis on its complex with SV40 T Ag; and to relate our work to that of others in the field. Finally, we will present the important questions arising from our work.

DISCOVERY AND DETECTION

Coprecipitation with Large T Ag

Immunoprecipitation of radiolabeled extracts of SV40-transformed or -infected cells, using serum from animals bearing SV40-induced tumors, followed by SDS-PAGE and fluorography, reveals, in addition to the viral large and small T antigens, the presence of a spectrum of bands with electrophoretic mobilities corresponding to apparent molecular weights in the range 48 to 55K daltons (Fig. 1) (2,5,10,18,19,22,27,28,36). The distribution and intensity of these bands is constant and characteristic of the cell line (28). The SV40-transformed mouse line SVA31E7 has only one readily detectable band, which we have characterized as 48K (2,28) and others have estimated as 53K (15,19,26) hence the term "p53," which is apparently becoming the consensus term for this class of polypeptides. Therefore the 48K in our figures is the same polypeptide as the consensus p53.

The host proteins can be readily labeled with a variety of radioactive amino acids. Although the most common practice is to use ^{35}S-methionine, the proteins have a very high relative content of arginine. All of the 48K–55K polypeptide species or subspecies can be radiolabeled with ^{32}P-orthophosphate (Fig. 1, right), indicating the protein(s) is a phosphoprotein.

Detecting Antibodies and Sera

The host proteins can be detected by "tumor sera" from hamsters or mice bearing SV40-induced tumors as previously noted. Monospecific antibodies prepared against SDS-PAGE-purified large T Ag immunoprecipitated the host proteins (2,19,28) leading Lane and Crawford (19) to recognize that the host protein is complexed to large T Ag.

Using SDS-PAGE, similar proteins were discovered in other systems, such as murine embryonal carcinoma cells (not infected by SV40) using immunoprecipitation by anti-SV40 tumor serum (22).

In a completely different system, i.e., in mice immunized with methylcholanthrene-induced tumors, a serum was obtained which immunoprecipitated the same proteins not only in the immunizing cells but also from cells transformed by the RNA tumor virus, murine sarcoma virus, and SV40 (7,16,17). The host protein "p50" was demonstrated in Abelson acute leukemia virus-transformed cells (33) and subsequently shown to be the same as those in SV40- and methylcholanthrene-transformed cells (33). Monospecific sera (26,27,29) and monoclonal antibodies (6,8,15) that recognize these host proteins have been prepared.

Homology of the Host Nuclear Phosphoproteins Among Mammalian Species

Two lines of evidence, one protein-chemical and the other immunological, indicate the host protein has both species-specific primary structure and, therefore, antigenic determinants, in addition to primary structure and antigenic determinants shared among species. The patterns of partial proteolysis fragments of the "48K" host nuclear phosphoprotein from mouse, hamster, and human cells is illustrated in Fig. 2 (27,29). It can be seen that there are both shared and unique proteolysis products indicating both shared and unique primary structure. This has also been reported by Simmons (35) using both partial proteolysis and tryptic fingerprinting.

The monospecific rabbit antibody against the SDS-PAGE-purified mouse 48K host protein is largely mouse-specific, having some slight reactivity against hamster and rat proteins, and none at all against those of monkey and human cells (27,29). On the other hand, the clone 122 mouse hybridoma of Gurney et al. (15), which recognizes the p53 and also recognizes our 48K host nuclear phosphoprotein complexed to SV40 T Ag (3), recognizes a determinant shared by the host proteins of all of the various mammalian species. The monoclonal antibody of Dippold et al. (8) recognizes both the mouse and human proteins. The fact that all of the mammalian species express a homologous protein(s) in response to SV40 infection or transformation argues for a shared response to the virus.

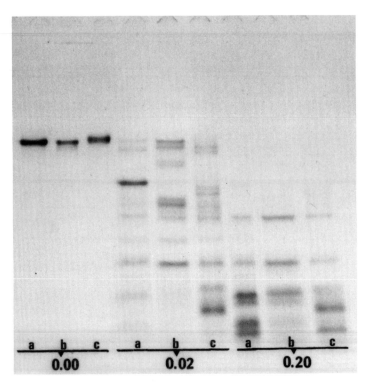

FIG. 2. Comparison of the partial digests of 48K host proteins isolated from cells of different mammalian species. The 48K host proteins were isolated and processed as described in Fig. 6. *a*, 48K protein of SV3T3 mouse cell; *b*, 48K host protein of SV28 hamster cells; *c*, 48K protein of SV80 human cells.

Molecular Weight Heterogeneity Within One Cell Type

As illustrated in Fig. 1, the host protein is heterogenous, with polypeptides we have estimated by Fergeson plots to be within the range Mr = 48 to 55K (28) and by others by SDS-PAGE mobility to be 44 to 60K (22), 50 to 60K (18), 50 to 55K (36), and 51 to 56 K (15), with p53 a more or less median value. We find (Fig. 1) on long 7.5 to 10% SDS-polyacrylamide gradient gels that there are two sets of doublets, one at about 48 to 50K, the other at about 52 to 55K. The 48 and 55K polypeptides are apparently different gene products with entirely different primary structures (27–29,39). There is further heterogeneity within the 48 to 50K and 52 to 55K families. We find the 48 to 50K polypeptide increases in mobility between a short pulse and a subsequent chase (R. B. Carroll, *unpublished observations*). The 48K host protein is also very heterogeneous on isoelectric focusing due to differential phosphorylation (3). Keeping this heterogeneity in mind, we will return to a discussion of the host proteins in the singular as is customary in this field.

Nuclear Localization

Using monospecific rabbit serum prepared against the mouse 48K host protein, we have shown it to have the same nuclear extranu-cleolar localization as that of SV40 large T Ag (27,29) (Fig. 3). This localization in SV40-transformed cells has been confirmed by others using a similar monospecific serum (26) and using mono-clonal sera (8,15). Figure 4 illustrates the same nuclear localization of the host protein in EBV-transformed cells using the serum from mice bearing the clone 122 hybridoma, carried out in collaboration with Dr. E. Gurney. This may be the same protein previously iso-lated by Luka et al. (24) in association with the Epstein Barr Virus Nuclear Antigen. Dippold et al. (8), using a monoclonal antibody against the mouse host protein, have found nuclear fluorescence in mouse cells transformed by methylcholanthrene, SV40, Moloney and Kirsten MuLVs, and X-rays, whereas in nontransformed mouse cells they found none. Using the same monoclonal anti-mouse host protein they reported immunofluorescence in the nuclei of dividing normal human kidney cells, and none in the nondividing cells. The nuclear localization of the 48K host protein suggests a nuclear func-tion, perhaps in the control of gene expression or replication.

Alternative localizations have been found for the 48K host pro-tein(s). A fraction of the host protein in wild-type SV40-transformed cells may be isolated from the plasma membrane and cytoplasmic fractions (20,21,37). Using the monoclonal antibody 2C2, which precipitates the p50, Coffman and Weissman (6) have obtained external plasma membrane fluorescence on normal and Abelson MuLV-transformed murine B cells, but not on normal T cells. Con-

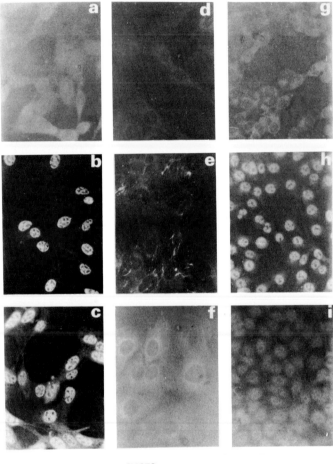

a SV 3T3
d 3T3
g SV 28

FIG. 3. Nuclear localization of the 48K host protein by indirect immunofluorescence. **a:** SV-BALB/c-3T3 cells vs normal rabbit serum. **b:** SV-BALB/c-3T3 cells vs rabbit anti-94K T Ag serum. **c:** SV-BALB/c-3T3 cells vs rabbit anti-48K serum. **d:** BALB/c-3T3 cells vs normal rabbit serum. **e:** BALB/c-3T3 cells vs rabbit anti-94K T Ag serum. **f:** BALB/c-3T3 cells vs rabbit anti-48K serum. **g:** SV28 cells vs normal rabbit serum. **h:** SV28 cells vs rabbit anti-94K T Ag serum. **i:** SV28 cells vs rabbit anti-48K serum.

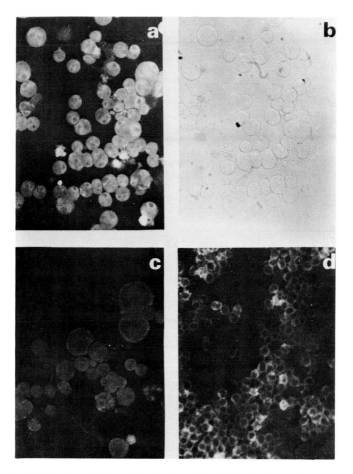

FIG. 4. Nuclear localization of the host protein in Epstein-Barr virus-transformed human cells. **a:** Raji cells were stained by indirect immunofluorescence using clone 122 hybridoma serum (15). **b:** The same field by light microscopy. **c:** Raji cells stained with normal mouse serum. **d:** Normal human lymphocytes stained with clone 122 hybridoma serum.

ventional anti-p50-reactive anti-tumor serum, which can immuno-precipitate the p50, also binds to the surface of Abelson-transformed cells (33). These results have strongly suggested the host protein can also be present at the plasma membrane. Using the clone 122 monoclonal antibody, we have found the host protein of the methylcholanthrene-transformed Balb/c line, Meth A, to occur in both nucleus and cytoplasm.

These various results indicate that the localization of the host protein is not entirely nuclear. Perhaps the host protein is found associated with the plasma membrane in nondividing normal cells, such as is the case with the B lymphocytes (6), but migrates to the nucleus before S phase, in order to trigger cell division.

Kinetics of Nuclear Appearance

The 48K host protein appears in the nucleus simultaneously with T Ag, 18 to 24 hr after infection of nonpermissive mouse cells with SV40 and before transformation (4) (Fig. 5). It had previously been shown the two polypeptides could be detected simultaneously in whole cell extracts (23). These results allow the possibility that formation of the 48K host protein-T Ag complex may be a necessary precondition for transformation. Our results (4) indicated, however, that essentially all the infected nonpermissive cells expressed both antigens (Fig. 5), whereas very few of the cells go on to be transformed, but instead revert to normal (i.e., are abortively transformed). This indicates that whereas the expression of the host protein and the formation of its complex with T Ag may be necessary for transformation, they are not sufficient for transformation. Per-

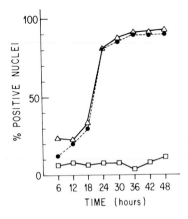

FIG. 5. Coordinate expression of the 48K host protein and SV40 large T Ag in nonpermissive cells. BALB/c 3T3 cells were infected, fixed, stained, and visualized as indicated in the text. Percentage of cells with positive nuclei staining with anti-94K large T Ag serum *(open triangles)*, anti-48K serum *(closed circles)*, and normal serum *(open squares)*. (From ref. 4, with permission.)

haps this is due to the fact that T Ag itself does not continue to be expressed in the abortively transformed cells. We will return to the question of involvement of the complex in transformation in the section on the effects of A locus mutation.

THE COMPLEX

Kinetics of Formation

To determine the kinetics of T Ag-48K host protein complex formation, a time course study was performed (13). Three identical cultures of SVA31E7 cells were labeled with [^{35}S] methionine: from 22 to 3 hr prior to harvest (long label); from 2.5 to 0.5 hr prior to harvest (intermediate label); and for 30 min prior to harvest (pulse). Thus, each of the three cultures had the same content of T Ag and concentration effects on the association were avoided. The extracts were then centrifuged on three parallel gradients and the distributions of antigens on the three gradients were compared after immuno-precipitation using a monospecific anti-94K T Ag serum (Fig. 6). It can be seen that with increasing time of labeling there is a progressive increase in the S value of T Ag, with the major distribution of T Ag occurring in fractions equivalent to 5 to 6S with a 30-min pulse (Fig. 6A), 15 to 16S after 3 hr (Fig. 6B), and 24S after 22 hr (Fig. 6C). However, the 48K host protein appears at high S values even after a 30-min pulse. As it was precipitated with an antiserum monospecific to large T Ag, the 48 K host protein must join the complex rapidly, and must be complexed to T Ag synthesized prior to the pulse. This experiment has been repeated using the monoclonal anti-T Ag clone 412 and anti-p53 host protein clone 122 of Gurney et al. (15), the results of which again indicate the host protein joins the complex early and the T Ag joins it late (3). This suggests that the host protein is limiting and the T Ag is in excess. It is also consistent with the results of Oren et al. (31), indicating that T Ag causes the expression of the host protein at high levels through stabilization of the polypeptide. It is not known, however, where the complex is formed. It is our hypothesis that the

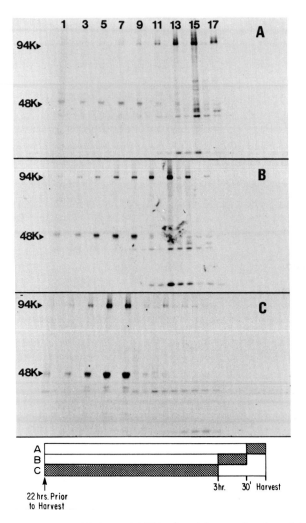

FIG. 6. Sedimentation of T Ag and 48K host protein as a function of duration of radiolabeling. Identical cultures of SVA31E7 cells were radiolabeled with [³⁵S]methionine for 30 min (150 μCi/ml in Dulbecco's modified Eagle's medium lacking methionine and containing 10% dialyzed calf serum), 2.5 hr (120 μCi/ml in Dulbecco's modified Eagle's medium containing 2% the normal concentration of methionine and 10% dialyzed calf serum), or 19.5 hr (20 μCi/ml in the same medium containing 10% the normal concentration of methionine and 10% dialyzed calf serum). The 2.5-hr and 19.5-hr radiolabeled cultures were then chased with complete Dulbecco's modified Eagle's medium containing 10% calf serum for 30 min and 3 hr, respectively. Cells were extracted and the extracts were sedimented on three parallel 5 to 20% sucrose gradients. Immunoprecipitation from gradient fractions was with hamster anti-tumor serum (odd numbered fractions) or normal hamster serum (even fractions). Autofluorograms are shown of the NaDodSO₄/7.5 to 15% polyacrylamide slab gel electrophoresis of fraction immunoprecipitates from gradients of 30-min pulse-labeled cells **(A)**, 2.5-hr-labeled cells chased for 30 min **(B)**, and 19.5-hr-labeled cells chased for 2.5 hr **(C)**.

complex is formed in the cytoplasm or at the plasma membrane and is then transported to the nucleus.

When [^{32}P]orthophosphate is used to radiolabel SVA31E7 cells using the same experimental protocol, a dramatically different result is obtained. The fluorograms at both the 30-min pulse and the 19-hr label with 3-hr chase look rather like Fig. 6B, suggesting phosphorylation of both "new" and "old" T Ags occurs. This is substantiated by the following experiment.

The 48K Host Protein Cosediments with Highly Phosphorylated T Ag

We have shown directly that T Ag is differentially phosphorylated (12). To examine the degree of phosphorylation of the multiple sedimenting forms of T Ag, an extract of SV40-transformed mouse cells (SVA31E7) radiolabeled with [^{3}H]methionine and [^{32}P]-orthophosphate was centrifuged on a 5 to 20% sucrose gradient (13). Immunoprecipitates of fractions from the gradient were then analyzed by NaDodSO$_4$/polyacrylamide gel electrophoresis and fluorography (Fig. 7A). The distribution of T Ag across the gradient is broad, as might be expected from an aggregating protein whose various aggregation states are in equilibrium with one another. It can be seen once again that the 48K host protein is detectable only in complexes with sedimentation coefficients of 16S or greater.

When the various bands of T Ag in Fig. 7A were excised and the ^{32}P and ^{3}H contents were determined, it was found that T Ag contained in complexes with sedimentation coefficients of 24S or greater had a higher ^{32}P/^{3}H ratio than any of the more slowly sedimenting forms (Fig. 7B and Table 1). Fraction 13 (15 to 16S), for example, has half the ^{32}P/^{3}H ratio of the 24S form. Comparison of the ^{32}P/^{3}H ratios of the various sedimenting forms of T Ag with the distribution of the 48K host protein on the same gradient (Fig. 7C) demonstrates that the host protein sediments predominantly with those forms of T Ag having the highest ^{32}P/^{3}H ratios. The relationship of ^{32}P/^{3}H ratios between the species of T Ag remains the same whether short (2 hr) or long (24 hr) periods of labeling are employed.

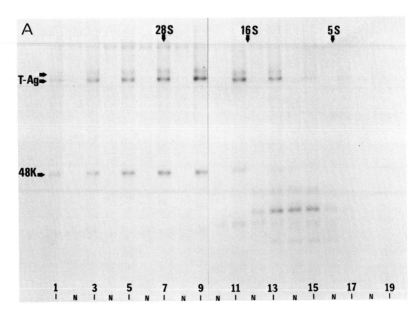

FIG. 7. Cosedimentation of the 48K host protein with the highly phosphorylated fraction of T Ag. SVA31E7 cells were labeled for 8 hr in Dulbecco's modified Eagle's medium containing 2% the normal concentrations of phosphate and methionine and 10% dialyzed calf serum with [^{32}P]orthophosphate at 320 μCi/ml and [^{3}H]methionine at 80 μCi/ml (New England Nuclear; 1 Ci = 3.7 × 10^{10} becquerels). Clarified extracts were then centrifuged through 5 to 20% sucrose gradients and fractions from these gradients were immunoprecipitated with hamster anti-tumor serum. **A:** Autofluorogram of NaDodSO$_4$/7.5 to 10% polyacrylamide slab gel electrophoresis of fraction immunoprecipitates. Columns labeled *N* and *I* correspond to samples immunoprecipitated with normal and immune hamster sera, respectively. *S* values were those of rRNA markers in a parallel gradient.

The ^{32}P/^{3}H ratio of the 24S species, for example, is always about twice that of the 15 to 16S form, which in turn is more than twice the ^{32}P/^{3}H ratio of T Ag sedimenting at 5 to 6S. This indicates that differences in ^{32}P/^{3}H ratios reflect differences in the phosphate content of protein species rather than differences in their rates of ^{32}P turnover. The ^{32}P/^{3}H ratios of the host protein in each of the fractions 3, 5, 7, and 9 were approximately equal and half that of the ^{32}P/^{3}H ratio of T Ag in the same fractions. ^{32}P/^{3}H ratios of host protein declined slightly through fractions 11 and 13.

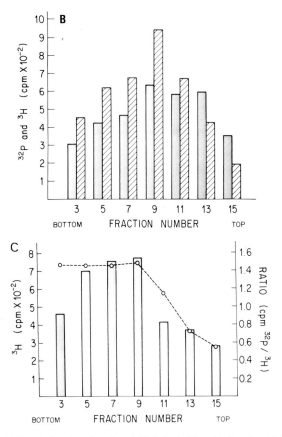

FIG. 7. *(contd.)* **B:** [32]P *(hatched bars)* and [3]H *(stippled bars)* in bands of 94,000 T Ag excised from the slab gel illustrated in **A. C:** [32]P/^{3}H ratios of T Ag bands in B (o---o) compared to ^{3}H in corresponding bands of 48K host protein from gel illustrated in **A.** Bottoms of gradients are to the left.

Phosphoserine and Phosphothreonine

As the form of T Ag which binds the 48K host protein is both the more highly phosphorylated and the less recently synthesized form, it is possible either that phosphorylation is essential to the complex formation or is incidental to it only reflecting the age of the T Ag. Our hypothesis was that a particular amino acid would

TABLE 1. *Ratios of 48K host protein/T Ag (as determined by*
[3]H contents) and ^{32}P/^{3}H ratios of doubly labeled T Ag and 48K
host protein in complexes of differing S values[a]

Fraction no.	[32]P/^{3}H, T Ag	[32]P/^{3}H, 48K host protein	48K host protein ^{3}H/T Ag[3]H
3	1.47	0.76	1.51
5	1.46	0.76	1.60
7	1.46	0.73	1.61
9	1.48	0.69	1.35
11	1.14	0.51	0.71
13	0.72	0.42	0.64
15	0.55		
17	0.43		

[a][32]P/[3]H = cpm[32]P/cpm[3]H. Bands were excised from the gel of
Fig. 7A and counted for ^{32}P,[3]H.

be phosphorylated in the complexed T Ag. To test the hypothesis,
we compared the ratio of phosphoserine and phosphothreonine in
T Ag at different periods of radiolabeling with [^{32}P]orthophosphate,
comparing the different sedimenting forms of T Ag, and comparing
the ratios after pulse and chases. Figure 8 illustrates the separation
we obtained between phosphoserine and phosphothreonine from
acid-hydrolysed fractions of T Ag, with hydrolysates from the top,
middle, and bottom of the gradient. When the phosphoamino acids
were scraped and counted, the results in Table 2 were obtained. No
significant difference in the ratio of the two amino acids was detected. Table 3 presents the results of an experiment designed to
determine whether phosphoserine and phosphothreonine have different turnover rates. Again, no difference could be detected. Thus,
at this point, we have no evidence suggesting that phosphoserines
or phosphothreonines are preferentially made or cleaved as a function of time after synthesis of large T antigen.

We found 7 to 8% of the phosphate in the 48K host protein of
SVA31E7 to be in the form of phosphothreonine, 91 to 93% in the
form of phosphoserine, and none as phosphotyrosine (Table 3).

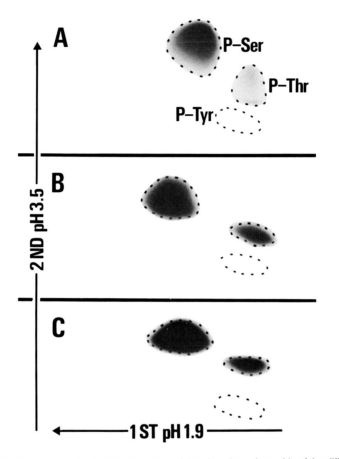

FIG. 8.   Two-dimensional electrophoresis of the phosphoamino acids of the different sedimenting forms of T Ag. Bands of T Ag were excised from an SDS-PAGE slab gel run as in Fig. 7. T Ag was then eluted and pooled in fractions representing rapidly sedimenting T Ag (columns 6 to 9), slowly sedimenting T Ag (columns 16 to 19), and T Ag of intermediate S values (columns 11 to 14). After precipitation in 20% TCA, the various forms of T Ag were subjected to acid hydrolysis in 6N HC1 at 110° C for 2 hr. HCl was then removed under reduced pressure and hydrolysates dissolved in a marker-mixture containing phosphoserine, phosphothreonine, and phosphotyrosine standards. Electrophoresis at pH 1.9 (first dimension) was for 3.5 hr at 400V in acetic acid/formic acid/H_2O, 25:78:897. Electrophoresis at pH 3.5 (second dimension), at right angles to the first dimension, was for 2 hr at 400V in pyridine/acetic acid/H_2O, 5:50:945. *Dashed circles* show positions of ninhydrin-stained phosphoamino acid markers. **A:** Slowly sedimenting T Ag. **B:** T Ag of intermediate S values. **C:** Rapidly sedimenting T Ag.

TABLE 2. *Quantitation of phosphoserine and phosphothreonine in the sedimenting forms of T Ag[a]*

T Ag size-class	Phosphoserine	Phosphothreonine
Top (fractions 16–19)	80.3% (1,708 cpm)	19.7% (418 cpm)
Middle (fractions 11–14)	76.1% (1,878 cpm)	23.9% (590 cpm)
Bottom (fractions 6–9)	80.3% (2,015 cpm)	19.7% (494 cpm)

[a]1×10^4 cpm of acid hydrolysate, in marker buffer, was applied to each of 3 thin layer plates. Approximately 25% of this was recovered as phosphoserine and phosphothreonine. The radioactivity in each phosphoamino acid is presented here as a percentage of the total radioactivity recovered as phosphoamino acids.

TABLE 3. *Results of an experiment on turnover rates and phosphoserine and phosphothreonine*

1 hr	Phosphorylated amino acid	CPM	Percent
94 pulse	p.ser.	1,400	70
	p.thr.	620	30
94 pulse/4-hr chase	p.ser.	1,150	61
	p.thr.	750	39
94 pulse/12-hr chase	p.ser.	765	73
	p.thr.	290	27
48 pulse	p.ser.	1,320	91.5
	p.thr.	122	8.5
48 pulse/4-hr chase	p.ser.	900	91.3
	p.thr.	86	8.7
48 pulse/12-hr chase	p.ser.	1,100	93
	p.thr.	77	7

VIRAL A LOCUS MUTATION

Mutation of the T Ag-encoding SV40 A locus leads to inhibition of viral replication in permissive cells and transformation of non-permissive cells (1,25,46). To implicate the 48K host nuclear phosphoprotein and its complex with T Ag in the transforming activity of T Ag, we sought to show an effect of A locus mutation on these biochemical activities. Nonpermissive Balb/c 3T3 cells were infected with either wild-type or tsA 58 SV40 at an m.o.i. = 200. Half of the tsA and wild-type SV40-infected cultures were maintained for 32 hr at the nonpermissive temperature of 39.5° C; the other half were maintained for 48 hr at the permissive temperature of 33° C. Cells were fixed and stained with monospecific anti-94K T Ag serum or with monospecific anti-48K host protein serum, with both sera or with rabbit prebleed serum. The percentage of positively stained nuclei at both temperatures with both viruses was determined. The results are shown in Fig. 9 (4). The data show that the percentage of T Ag and 48K host protein-positive cells in a tsA-infected culture at the nonpermissive temperature is approximately 19% of that at the permissive temperature. In both cases the percentage of T Ag or 48K host protein positive cells was equal to those stained with both sera, indicating that in both cases the 48K host protein and T Ag were expressed in the same cells. The percentage of T Ag and 48K host protein-positive cells in wild type-infected cultures was the same at either temperature. We interpret the data to mean that the tsA mutant is slightly "leaky" at the nonpermissive temperature with the high multiplicities of infection we were obliged to use, due to the refractory nature of BALB/c 3T3 cells to infection by SV40. A few cells produced enough stable T Ag to stain with anti-94K serum. Those few cells that produced

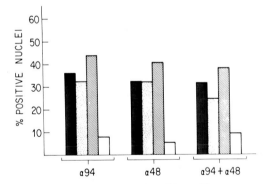

FIG. 9. A locus dependence of the expression of the 48K host tumor antigen. BALB/c 3T3 cells were infected with either wild-type (WT) or tsA58 (tsA) virus as indicated in the text. Indirect immunofluorescent staining was performed using either anti-94K large T Ag serum, anti-48K serum, both sera together, or normal serum (not shown). *Hatched bars*, WT 33° C; *speckled bars*, WT 39.5° C; *stippled bars*, tsA 33° C; *open bars*, tsA 39.5° C. (From ref. 4, with permission.)

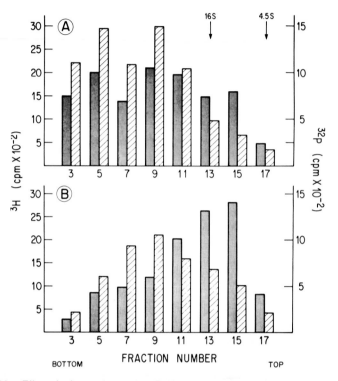

FIG. 10. Effect of tsA mutation on the ^{32}P/^{3}H-labeled complexes. TsA 58-transformed mouse embryo fibroblasts maintained at 33° C or shifted to 39.5° C were labeled with both [^{3}H]methionine (107 μCi/ml) and [^{32}P]orthophosphate (428 μCi/ml) at either 33° C or 39.5° C (15 hr after shift-up). After centrifugation of extracts through parallel 5 to 20% sucrose gradients and immunoprecipitation of fractions with monospecific rabbit antiserum to 94,000 T Ag and subsequent NaDodSO$_4$/polyacrylamide gel electrophoresis, the T Ag and 48K host protein were excised from the slab gels, and ^{32}P *(hatched bars)* and ^{3}H *(stippled bars)* contents were determined. **A:** T Ag radiolabeled at 33° C. **B:** T Ag radiolabeled at 39.5° C.

detectable T Ag also produced the 48K host protein. Using an immunoprecipitation assay, Linzer et al. (23) had shown an A Locus-dependence of the expression of the host protein.

To determine the effect of the small t Ag locus on the induction of the 48K host protein, we infected cultures of Balb/c 3T3 cells with two different deletion mutants that produce a functionally defective small t Ag: dl 884, which is missing the sequence from 0.54

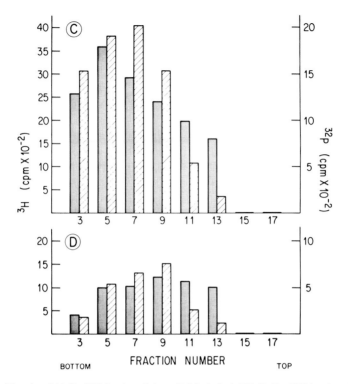

FIG. 10. *(contd.)* **C:** 48K host protein radiolabeled at 33° C. **D:** 48K host protein radiolabeled at 39.5° C. S values were those of bovine serum albumin (4.5S); and β-galactosidase (16S). The bottoms of the gradients are to the left.

to 0.58, and dl 890, deleted from 0.58 to 0.59 on the genome (34). The fixed and stained cells showed that the 48K host protein is still induced by these deletion mutants. It is clear from these results that the expression of the 48K host protein is dependent on the A locus and is independent of the region 0.54 to 0.59, which encodes part of small t Ag but does not encode large T Ag.

We have also examined the effect of the mutation on the formation of the 48K host protein-T Ag complex. Using tsA 58-transformed mouse cells radiolabeled either singly with [^{35}S]methionine or doubly with [^{3}H]methionine and [^{32}P]orthophosphate, we have shown the mutant T Ag is inhibited in its ability to complex the 48K host protein and to associate beyond the 5 to 6S monomer (13).

To determine whether the predominantly 5 to 6S species of monomeric T Ag generated in tsA-transformed cells at the nonpermissive temperature is also minimally phosphorylated, tsA 58-transformed cells were radiolabeled with both [³H]methionine and [³²P]orthophosphate at either the permissive or nonpermissive temperature. Immunoprecipitation from gradients was performed with antiserum to 94K T Ag. Bands of T Ag and 48K host protein, located in subsequent NaDodSO₄/polyacrylamide slab gels by fluorography, were then excised and ³H and ³²P contents were measured. In Fig. 10A, it can be seen that T Ag radiolabeled at the permissive temperature is found predominantly as rapidly sedimenting, highly phosphorylated species. T Ag radiolabeled at the nonpermissive temperature (Fig. 10B), however, sediments predominantly as a 5 to 6S monomeric form (fraction 15). In addition, this species of T Ag was minimally phosphorylated, whereas the small percentage of T Ag remaining complexed to 48K host protein at the nonpermissive temperature was phosphorylated to the same extent as the T Ag in complexes of similar S values at the permissive temperature. This implies a close and perhaps causal relationship between the phosphorylation state of T Ag and its ability to complex 48K host protein.

It can be seen that there is much less of the 48K host protein complexed to T Ag at the nonpermissive temperature (Fig. 10D) than at the permissive temperature (Fig. 10C). It is striking that although the total [³H]methionine in T Ag at the nonpermissive temperature is 93% that of T Ag at the permissive temperature, the total [³H]methionine in the 48K host protein at the nonpermissive temperature is only 38% of that of 48K host protein at the permissive temperature. The overall ³²P/³H ratio of the 48K host protein is the same at both the permissive and nonpermissive temperatures, in contrast to the effect on T Ag.

These results show that A locus mutation inhibits the ability of T Ag to complex the host protein and to become maximally phosphorylated. This strongly suggests a role for the host protein in the activity of T Ag and, therefore, in transformation by SV40.

DNA BINDING

As the 48K host protein both complexes T Ag and is found *in vivo* in the nucleus, it is then likely that it binds with T Ag to the cellular DNA. To test this, SVA31E7 cells were radiolabeled with [^{35}S]methionine, and the T Ag-48K host protein complex partially purified by nuclear preparation, ammonium sulfate fractionation, and DEAE cellulose column chromatography (27). The protein was then applied to a calf thymus double-stranded DNA cellulose column. The column was washed and then eluted with high salt buffer. Figure 11 shows that the 48K host protein was immunoprecipitable with T Ag in the high salt eluate, indicating it bound with T Ag to DNA (27).

To determine whether T Ag subfractions differing in their affinities for host chromatin differed in their ^{32}P/^{3}H ratios, SVA31E7 cells were again double labeled with [^{3}H]methionine and [^{32}P]orthophosphate. The nuclei of these cells were then isolated and serially extracted with buffers of increasing pH. The various extraction supernatants were then immunoprecipitated with hamster anti-tumor serum and the immunoprecipitates were separated by NaDodSO$_4$/polyacrylamide gel electrophoresis (Fig. 12A). It can be seen that both T Ag and the 48K host protein eluted from host chromatin at pH 7.0, 8.0, and 9.0 but not at pH 6.0 (13). Small amounts of both proteins were found in the cytoplasmic faction and may have eluted from nuclei under the conditions employed for nuclear isolation. Determination of ^{32}P and ^{3}H contents in the various fractions of T Ag revealed that although the major fraction of T Ag eluted at pH 8.0, T Ag eluting at pH 9.0 contained the most phosphate. The ^{32}P/^{3}H ratio of T Ag increased with its affinity for host chromatin (Fig. 12B). This result is in agreement with the results of Montenarh and Henning (30), who compared the phosphorylation of T Ag fractions eluting from DNA cellulose, and found the more tightly bound T Ag to be the more phosphorylated.

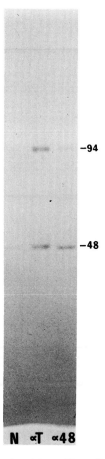

FIG. 11. Binding of the 48K host protein and large T antigen to calf thymus double-stranded DNA cellulose. The 17 to 45% saturated ammonium sulfate fraction of an extract of [35S]methionine-labeled SV3T3 cells was applied to calf thymus double-stranded DNA cellulose. The pH 8.0 eluate was immunoprecipitated using normal *(N)*, anti-T *(αT)*, or anti-48K serum *(α48)*. The immunoprecipitates were subjected to SDS-PAGE and visualized by fluorography.

MODEL OF COMPLEX FORMATION

Our work indicates that a sequence of reactions takes place between T Ag and the 48K host nuclear phosphoprotein, involving phosphorylation of T Ag and leading to subsequent multimeric association and chromatin binding by the T Ag-48K host protein complexes. This reaction sequence is schematized in Fig. 13.

Reactions 1 and 2: Phosphorylation and 48K Host Protein Binding

The close, perhaps causal, relationship between the level of phosphorylation of T Ag and its ability to complex 48K host protein suggests two possibilities: pathway A, progressive phosphorylation of T Ag enhances its binding affinity for 48K host protein or pathway B, T Ag must first be complexed to 48K host protein for maximal phosphorylation to occur. The minimal phosphorylation of monomeric T Ag is rapid, whereas the progressive phosphorylation accompanying complex formation with the 48K host protein is slow. This might suggest that two different functional types of phosphate exist on the T Ag molecule. However, our results indicate that the ratio of phosphoserine to phosphothreonine is uniform throughout the gradient but that an increase in total phosphorylation correlates with aggregation. It may also be that the maximal phosphorylation of T Ag has no relation to the complex formation but is a product of changed intracellular localization of the complex.

The ability of tsA locus mutations to inhibit both the phosphorylation of T Ag and its ability to complex the 48K host protein indicates that these activities may be important in affecting one or more functions of the A locus.

Reaction 3: Association to Multimers

The smallest T Ag-48K host protein complexes sediment at 15 to 16S; T Ag in these complexes is half as phosphorylated as the maximally phosphorylated T Ag of larger complexes. The smallest complexes containing maximally phosphorylated T Ag sediment at 24S. In addition to containing T Ag twice as phosphorylated as that in the 15 to 16S complex, the 24S complex has twice the ratio of 48K host protein to T Ag as the 15 to 16S form. Multimeric complexes sedimenting faster than 24S have the same ratio of 48K host protein to T Ag and contain T Ag phosphorylated to the same extent as in the 24S form. Ratios of 48K host protein to T Ag are the same whether immunoprecipitations are performed with antitumor or monospecific anti-94K T Ag serum. This indicates that the ratios are those of true complexes and are not derived from cosedimentation of homopolymers of T Ag and the host protein.

In time course studies, monomeric T Ag appears as a significant fraction of T Ag in cells transformed by wild-type SV40 only on labeling for short periods of time (Fig. 6A). The conversion of minimally phosphorylated, monomeric T Ag to more highly phosphorylated, complexed forms, therefore, either is unidirectional or involves an equilibrium strongly favoring formation of highly phosphorylated complexed T Ag. We have found that the maximally phosphorylated species of T Ag in rapidly sedimenting complexes ($\geq$ 24S) contains about 4 times the phosphate of monomeric T Ag. Walter and Flory (47) have determined that T Ag of SV40-infected cells contains an average of four phosphates per molecule. Our results are, therefore, consistent with the existence of highly phosphorylated T Ag in high molecular weight complexes, which represent the predominant form of T Ag in SV40-transformed cells and have three to four phosphates per molecule.

Reaction 4: Chromatin Binding

T Ag binds DNA in the absence of other proteins (38,43). It has yet to be determined whether the host protein can bind DNA in the absence of T Ag. However, the finding that the most phosphorylated form of T Ag both complexes the host protein and binds with greatest affinity to host chromatin suggests that high molecular weight T Ag-48K host protein complexes represent the major form of T Ag bound to host chromatin *in vivo*. This hypothesis is supported by immunofluorescence studies in which T Ag and 48K host protein were found to have the same distribution in the nuclei of SV40-transformed cells (27). Moreover, T Ag and the host protein have been shown to co-chromatograph, as complexes, on DNA-cellulose columns (27). Other groups have reported that tsA lesions impair the ability of T Ag to bind host chromatin (41) and SV40 DNA (42). We propose this may result from a prior effect of the tsA lesion on the phosphorylation of T Ag and its ability to complex the host proteins (reactions 1 and 2, Fig. 13). Thus, tsA inhibition of the phosphorylation of T Ag and its ability to complex the host protein would interfere with A locus functions requiring the complex to interact with host chromatin, including initiation of replication, and establishment and maintenance of viral transformation.

FUTURE QUESTIONS

Our present hypothesis is that the 48K host protein or p53 is involved in triggering the S phase leading to cell division and that the viral T Ag subverts the triggering mechanism from within the cell. We think SV40 T Ag binds to the host enzymes involved in cellular replication and that the 48K host protein is the first of these proteins to be isolated and identified in the complex. One of the primary characteristics of transformed cells is that they have lost many of the normal controls to cell division. SV40 can induce quiescent cells to divide (46), evidently through the activity of large T Ag. The wide distribution of the host protein in the nuclei of cells transformed by a variety of agents (4,8,15,27,29) fits this hypothesis. We might expect a molecule involved in triggering cell division to be a membrane protein, which is responsive to external growth factors, and which migrates to the nucleus to trigger S phase. There are suggestions that the 48K host protein may also be found at the plasma membrane (6,32,37). Our hypothesis would then require T Ag to complex the host protein at the plasma membrane. It is not known at present whether either T Ag or the host protein are made on the rough endoplasmic reticulum or on free polysomes. Nor is it known whether either goes to the plasma membrane when first synthesized, or whether either goes straight to the nucleus. We have shown that the complex can be detected in the cytoplasm, and,

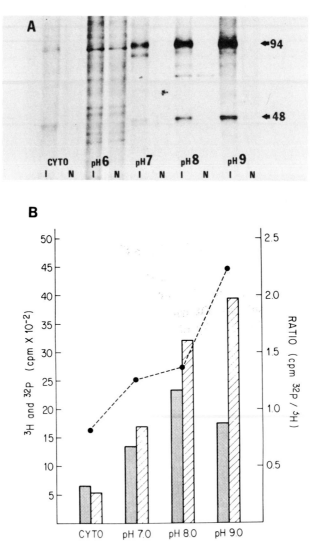

FIG. 12. [32]P/^{3}H ratios of different chromatin-binding forms of T Ag. SVA31E7 cells starved for 1 hr in Dulbecco's modified Eagle's medium minus methionine and phosphate and containing 10% dialyzed calf serum were labeled for 3.5 hr with 200 μCi of [^{32}P]orthophosphate per ml and 50 μCi of [^{3}H]methionine per ml. Cell nuclei were then isolated and serially extracted with pH 6.0, 7.0, 8.0, and 9.0 buffers and then immunoprecipitated. **A:** Autofluorogram of NaDodSO$_4$/7.5 to 15% polyacrylamide slab gel electrophoresis. Immunoprecipitations were with hamster anti-tumor serum *(I)* or normal hamster serum *(N)*. **B:** Samples larger than those applied to the slab gel in **A** were electrophoresed in cylindrical NaDodSO$_4$/8.5% polyacrylamide gels. These gels were then sliced and the [32]P *(hatched bars)* and [3]H *(stippled bars)* in the various peaks of T Ag were determined. The background from parallel gels run with normal precipitates has been subtracted. (o---o) ^{32}P/^{3}H ratios. *Cyt*, cytoplasmic fraction.

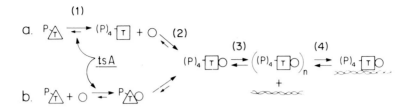

FIG. 13. Proposed reaction sequence for T Ag-48K host protein-DNA interactions affected by the phosphorylation of T Ag. *Triangles*, minimally phosphorylated molecules of T Ag. *Squares*, maximally phosphorylated molecules of T Ag. *Circles*, the 48K host protein (p53). *Double helix*, double-stranded DNA. See text for discussion.

therefore, the complex can evidently form before reaching the nucleus. We also have to explain the peculiarly slow kinetics with which newly synthesized large T Ag joins the complex with the host protein. Could this be due to a limiting concentration of the host protein or to a difference in compartmentalization of the free and bound T Ag? Another corollary of the hypothesis is that although the host protein is present in the nuclei of transformed cells throughout the cell cycle, it should be present in the plasma membranes but absent from the nuclei of normal cells except in the S phase.

What is its molecular function or enzymatic activity? There are three slightly suggestive bits of evidence that the host protein may be a protein kinase: (a) a protein kinase co-purifies with T Ag (14,44) but is separable from T Ag (11,45); (b) maximal phosphorylation of T Ag is associated with complex formation (9,13); and (c) it has been shown recently that a protein kinase is associated with the host protein immunoprecipitated from Meth A cells by a monoclonal antibody (17). Nothing is firmly established, however, about the activity, substrate, or biological activity of the 48K host protein.

Finally, it is of interest to determine (a) if the host protein is the only product to complex with T Ag or if, on the contrary, other polypeptides are to be discovered in the complex, and (b) the link between transformation by the RNA and DNA tumor viruses implied by the presence of the same host protein in cells transformed by both classes of agent.

ACKNOWLEDGMENTS

We thank Ms. Joni Hart for typing this manuscript. This work was supported by U.S. Public Health Service grants 5 T32 CA9161 and CA 20802 and CA 16329. The first author is a Scholar of the Leukemia Society of America. This work was performed in facilities provided by the New York University Cancer Center.

REFERENCES

1. Carroll, R. B., and Defendi, V. (1981): Viral nuclear antigens. In: *Biochemistry and Biology of the Cell Nucleus*, edited by L. Hnilica. CRC Press Cleveland *(in press)*.
2. Carroll, R. B., Goldfine, S. 2M., and Melero, J. A. (1978): Antiserum to polyacrylamide gel-purified simian virus 40 T antigen. *Virology*, 87:194–198.
3. Carroll, R. B., and Gurney, E. G. (1982): *Submitted for publication*.
4. Carroll, R. B., Muello, K., and Melero, J. A. (1980): Coordinate expression of the 48K host nuclear phosphoprotein and SV40 T Ag upon primary infection of mouse cells. *Virology*, 102:447–452.
5. Chang, C., Simmons, D. T., Martin, M. A., and Mora, P. T. (1979): Identification and partial characterization of new antigens from simian virus 40-transformed mouse cells. *J. Virol.*, 31:463–471.
6. Coffman, R. L., and Weissman, I. L. (1981): A monoclonal antibody which recognizes B cells and B cell precursors in mice. *J. Exp. Med.*, 153:269–279.
7. DeLeo, A. B., Jay, G., Apella, E., Dubois, G. C., Law, L. W., and Old, L. J. (1979): Detection of a transformation-related antigen in chemically induced sarcomas and other transformed cells of the mouse. *Proc. Natl. Acad. Sci. USA*, 76:2420–2424.
8. Dippold, W. G., Jay, G., DeLeo, A. B., Khoury, G., and Old, L. J. (1981): p53 transformation-related protein: Detection by monoclonal antibody in mouse and human cells. *Proc. Natl. Acad. Sci. USA*, 78:1695–1699.
9. Fanning, E., Nowak, B., and Burger, C. (1981): Detection and characterization of multiple forms of simian virus 40 large T antigen. *J. Virol.*, 37:92–102.
10. Gaudray, P., Rassoulzadegan, M., and Cuzin, F. (1978): Expression of simian virus 40 early genes in transformed rat cells is correlated with maintenance of the transformed phenotype. *Proc. Natl. Acad. Sci. USA*, 75:4987–4991.
11. Giacherio, D., and Hager, L. P. (1979): A poly(dT)-stimulated ATPase activity associated with simian virus 40 large T antigen. *J. Biol. Chem.*, 254:8113–8116.

12. Greenspan, D. S., and Carroll, R. (1979): Simian virus 40 large T antigen isoelectric focuses as multiple species with varying phosphate content. *Virology*, 99:413–416.
13. Greenspan, D. S., and Carroll, R. B. (1981): Complex of simian virus 40 large tumor antigen and 48,000-dalton host tumor antigen. *Proc. Natl. Acad. Sci. USA*, 78:105–109.
14. Griffin, J. D., Spangler, G., and Livingston, D. M. (1979): Enzymatic Activities Associated with the SV40 Large T Antigen. *Cold Spring Harbor Symp. Quant. Biol.*, 44:113–122.
15. Gurney, E. G., Harrison, R. O., and Fenno, J. (1980): Monoclonal antibodies against simian virus 40 T antigens: Evidence for distinct subclasses of large T antigen and for similarities among nonviral T antigens. *J. Virol.*, 34:752–763.
16. Jay, G., DeLeo, A. B., Apella, E., Dubois, G. C., Law, L. W., Khoury, G., and Old, L. J. (1979): A common transformation-related protein in murine sarcomas and leukemias. *Cold Spring Harbor Symp. Quant. Biol.*, 44:659–664.
17. Jay, G., Khoury, G., DeLeo, A. B., Dippold, W. G., and Old, L. J. (1981): p53 transformation-related protein: Detection of an associated phosphotransferase activity. *Proc. Natl. Acad. Sci. USA*, 78:2932–2936.
18. Kress, M., May, E., Cassingena, R., and May, P. (1979): Simian virus 40-transformed cells express new species of proteins precipitable by anti-simian virus 40 tumor serum. *J. Virol.*, 31:472–483.
19. Lane, D. P., and Crawford, L. V. (1979): T antigen is bound to a host protein in SV40-transformed cells. *Nature*, 278:261–263.
20. Lanford, R. E., and Butel, J. S. (1980): Inhibition of nuclear migration of wild-type SV40 tumor antigen by a transport-defective mutant of SV40-adenovirus 7 hybrid virus. *Virology*, 105:303–313.
21. Lanford, R. E., and Butel, J. S. (1980): Biochemical characterization of nuclear and cytoplasmic forms of SV40 tumor antigens encoded by parental and transport-defective mutant SV40-adenovirus 7 hybrid viruses. *Virology*, 105:314–327.
22. Linzer, D. I. H., and Levine, A. J. (1979): Characterization of a 54K dalton cellular SV40 tumor antigen present in SV40-transformed cells and uninfected embryonal carcinoma cells. *Cell*, 17:43–52.
23. Linzer, D. I. H., Maltzman, W., and Levine, A. J. (1979): The SV40: A gene product is required for the production of a 54,000 MW cellular tumor antigen. *Virology*, 98:308–318.
24. Luka, J., Jornval, H., and Klein, G. (1980): Purification and biochemical characterization of the Epstein-Barr virus-determined nuclear antigen and an associated protein with a 53,000-dalton subunit. *J. Virol.*, 35:592–602.
25. Martin, R. G. (1981): The transformation of cell growth and transmogrification of DNA synthesis by simian virus 40. *Adv. Cancer Res.*, 34:1–68.
26. McCormick, F., and Harlow, E. (1980): Association of a murine 53,000-dalton phosphoprotein with simian virus 40 large-T antigen in transformed cells. *J. Virol.*, 34:213–224.

27. Melero, J. A., Greenspan, D. S., and Carroll, R. B. (1979): T-antigen-associated protein induced by SV40 transformation. *Cold Spring Harbor Symp. Quant. Biol.*, 44:201–209.

28. Melero, J. A., Stitt, D. T., Mangel, W. F., and Carroll, R. B. (1979): Identification of new polypeptide species (48–55K) immunoprecipitable by antiserum to purified large T antigen and present in SV40-infected and -transformed cells. *Virology*, 93:466–480.

29. Melero, J. A., Tur, S., and Carroll, R. B. (1980): Host nuclear proteins expressed in simian virus 40-transformed and -infected cells. *Proc. Natl. Acad. Sci. USA*, 77:97–101.

30. Montenarh, M., and Henning, R. (1980): Simian virus 40 T antigen phosphorylation is variable. *FEBS Lett.*, 114:107–110.

31. Oren, M., Maltzman, W., and Levine, A. J. (1981): Post-translational regulation of the 54K cellular tumor antigen in normal and transformed cells. *Mol. Cell. Biol.*, 1:101–110.

32. Rotter, V., Boss, M. A., and Baltimore, D. (1981): Increased concentration of an apparently identical cellular protein in cells transformed by either Abelson murine leukemia virus or other transforming agents. *J. Virol.*, 38:336–346.

33. Rotter, V., Witte, O. N., Coffman, R., and Baltimore, D. (1980): Abelson murine leukemia virus-induced tumors elicit antibodies against a host cell protein, p50. *J. Virol.*, 36:547–555.

34. Shenk, T. E., Carbon, J., and Berg, P. (1976): Construction and analysis of viable deletion mutants of simian virus 40. *J. Virol.*, 18:664–671.

35. Simmons, D. T. (1980): Characterization of T antigens isolated from uninfected and simian virus 40-transformed monkey cells and papovavirus-transformed cells. *J. Virol.*, 36:519–525.

36. Smith, A. E., Smith, R., and Paucha, E. (1979): Characterization of different tumor antigens present in cells transformed by simian virus 40. *Cell*, 18:335–336.

37. Soule, H. R., Lanford, R. E., and Butel, J. S. (1980): Antigenic and immunogenic characteristics of nuclear and membrane-associated simian virus 40 tumor antigen. *J. Virol.*, 33:887–901.

38. Spillman, T., Giacherio, D., and Hager, L. P. (1979): Single strand DNA binding of simian virus 40 tumor antigen. *J. Biol. Chem.*, 254:3100–3104.

39. Stitt, D. T., Carroll, R. B., Melero, J. A., and Mangel, W. F. (1981): Analysis of the 84K, 55K, and 48K proteins immunoprecipitable by SV40 T antibody from SV40-infected and -transformed cells by tryptic peptide mapping on cation-exchange columns. *Virology*, 111:283–288.

40. Tegtmeyer, P. (1972): Simian virus 40 deoxyribonucleic acid synthesis: The viral replicon. *J. Virol.* 10:591–598.

41. Tegtmeyer, P., Schwartz, M., Collins, J. K., and Rundell, K. (1975): Regulation of tumor antigen synthesis by simian virus 40 gene A. *J. Virol.*, 16:168–178.

42. Tenen, D. G., Baygell, P., and Livingston, D. M. (1975): Thermolabile T (tumor) antigen from cells transformed by a temperature-sensitive mutant of simian virus 40. *Proc. Natl. Acad. Sci. USA*, 72:4351–4355.
43. Tjian, R. (1978): Protein-DNA interactions at the origin of simian virus 40 DNA replication. *Cold Spring Harbor Symp. Quant. Biol.*, 43:655.
44. Tjian, R., and Robbins, A. (1979): Enzymatic activities associated with a purified simian virus 40 T antigen-related protein. *Proc. Natl. Acad. Sci. USA*, 76:610–614.
45. Tjian, R., Robbins, A., and Clark, R. (1979): Catalytic properties of the SV40 large T antigen. *Cold Spring Harbor Symp. Quant. Biol.*, 44:103–111.
46. Tooze, J., ed. (1980): *Part 2: DNA Tumor Viruses Molecular Biology of Tumor Viruses*. Cold Spring Harbor Laboratory, Cold Spring Harbor, New York.
47. Walter, G., and Flory, P. J. (1979): Phosphorylation of SV40 large T antigen. *Cold Spring Harbor Symp. Quant. Biol.*, 44:165–169.

Advances in Viral Oncology, Volume 2, edited by
George Klein. Raven Press, New York © 1982.

p53: A Transformation-Related Protein Found in Chemically Induced Sarcomas and Other Transformed Cells

*Ettore Appella and **Vincent J. Hearing

*Laboratory of Cell Biology and **Dermatology Branch, National Cancer
Institute, National Institutes of Health, Bethesda, Maryland 20205*

During the last few years, several cellular proteins that may play a role in the transformation of normal cells to malignancy have been characterized. The system most clearly characterized to date is that of the Rous (or avian) sarcoma virus. Normal cells contain a 60,000 dalton protein (pp60[sarc]) that is structurally related to the product of the oncogenic gene (pp60[src]) and is associated with protein kinase activity acting on tyrosine residues (3,4,26,28). The pp60[sarc] protein, which is present in normal cells in 30- to 50-fold lower concentrations than that of pp60[src] in transformed cells, may well be involved in some critical cellular function, such as maintenance of control over cell division. A second example of similarity between transforming proteins and normal components is found in Abelson virus-induced lymphomas. A normal 150,000 dalton cell component has been identified in thymus and other lymphoid organs; this protein shares common antigenic determinants with p120, which is a protein encoded by the Abelson MuLV genome (35). The 150,000 dalton normal cell protein occurs at concentrations much lower than its counterpart in virally transformed cells. These two examples demonstrate that present in the cell are genes that are not deleterious during normal expression, and may even be vital for normal growth and development. These genes have apparently been transduced by viruses and joined to regulatory elements that dramatically increase their rates of expression. The pleiotropic effects of these proteins on multiple target molecules in the cell may induce transformation.

One of the questions that has been raised is whether there are other proteins that may be involved in transformation, but are brought about by completely different mechanisms. The large T protein that is encoded by the early region of simian virus 40 (SV40) is involved in the induction and maintenance of cell transformation (22,33). To understand the mechanism of SV40-induced transformation, efforts have been initiated to determine how the large T protein interacts with components of the host cell. Early reports showed that the T antigen in a line of SV40-transformed mouse cells formed a complex with a specific, cell-coded 53,000 dalton protein (p53) (15). The molecular nature of this protein has now been further elucidated and, as shown later in this chapter, it seems to act as a regulator of certain cellular functions related to growth control, and its expression appears to be elevated in the transformed state.

DETECTION OF p53 ANTIGEN

The p53 antigen was initially detected by the use of an antiserum obtained from BALB/c or (BALB/c × C57BL/6)F$_1$ hybrid mice hyperimmunized with a syngeneic methylcholanthrene-induced sarcoma (Meth A) (6). Extracts of radiolabeled Meth A sarcoma cells were incubated with either the Meth A antiserum or normal murine serum. The resulting immune complexes were precipitated with protein A-bearing *Staphylococcus aureus* and analyzed by SDS polyacrylamide gel electrophoresis, followed by autoradiography. The results clearly established that the Meth A sarcoma cells synthesized a 53,000 dalton component (p53), which was apparently absent from normal BALB/c lung fibroblasts. Sera raised against 25 different tumor cell lines were tested for anti-p53 reactivity, and only a similarly prepared antiserum against a BALB/c sarcoma (CMS4) demonstrated anti-p53 activity (6). The basis for this difference is not yet known; it is possible that higher levels of p53 are expressed in certain tumors, or that an adjuvant effect of p53-associated proteins may play a role in the induction of antibody production.

Methylcholanthrene-induced sarcomas, however, were not the only tumor cells capable of eliciting antibody to p53. Sera obtained from either mice or hamsters bearing SV40-induced tumors (18,31), or Abelson-MuLV-induced lymphoid tumor cells (30), were also capable of precipitating p53 from extracts of Meth A and other transformed cell lines of the mouse.

A wide range of neoplastic cell lines of BALB/c origin that had been transformed by X-ray, viral, or chemical agents have been analyzed for the presence of p53 by immunoprecipitation. All the transformed cells tested had high titers of this antigen (11). Of all nontransformed cells tested, only normal thymocytes from 2- to 9-month-old mice had detectable amounts of p53, although the concentration was about 10-fold lower than that found in Meth A sarcoma cells.

Recently, monoclonal antibodies to p53 have been described. These antibodies have been prepared by fusion of spleen cells from mice that had been immunized with BALB/c methylcholanthrene-induced sarcoma, CMS4 (7), or SV40-transformed murine cells (9); monoclonal antibodies have also been prepared from rats that had been immunized with Abelson-MuLV-induced tumor cells (RAW12) (2). These reagents have confirmed the immunoprecipitation studies performed with antisera from tumor-bearing or immunized mice. In addition, these monoclonal antibodies detected a protein of approximately 53,000 daltons in certain spontaneously or *in vitro* SV40-transformed human cells (5). Investigations with these monoclonal antibodies have also been carried out to study the occurrence of p53 by indirect immunofluorescence (7). In agreement with the results of immunoprecipitation studies, immunofluorescence tests demonstrated the presence of p53 in all transformed murine cell lines previously examined (Table 1).

In addition, the intracellular location of p53 was examined. The fluorescence was primarily confined to the nucleus. The strength of the immunofluorescence reaction varied considerably; the SV40-transformed cells showed the strongest reaction and the leukemias, the weakest reaction (7). No p53 reactivity has been observed by immunofluorescence in a variety of normal murine cells, including

TABLE 1. *Survey of murine-transformed cell lines containing p53 detectable by immunofluorescence and immunoprecipitation*

Cell line	Transforming agent
Meth A, C1, C1-4, C2-10, CMS3, CMS4, CMS5, B6MS2 sarcomas	Methylcholanthrene
CTF sarcoma, F9 teratocarcinoma	Spontaneous
F9 12-1 clone	pBR322/HSV-1 tk/SV40 DNA
F9 12-1a clone	pBR322/HSV-1 tk/SV40 DNA treated with retinoic acid
3T3 WT sarcoma	SV40
11A sarcoma	Moloney MuSV
K234 sarcoma	Kirsten MuSV

normal adult BALB/c thymus. This result is in sharp contrast with the detection of p53 in extracts of thymus by immunoprecipitation with either conventional or monoclonal antibodies and can be attributed to the lower sensitivity of this method.

Unexpected and potentially interesting results have been obtained with a rat monoclonal antibody, RA3-2C2 (2,30). This reagent precipitated p53 from a variety of transformed cells. However, cell surface labeling has been found on an Abelson-MuLV lymphoma, 2M3, and on 20% of normal bone marrow cells. These normal cells appear to be early B-cells, i.e., surface immunoglobulin negative. This antibody does not surface label thymocytes, peripheral T cells, nonlymphoid hematopoietic cells in the spleen or bone marrow, or the hematopoietic stem cells. It appears, therefore, that exteriorization of this antigen is a characteristic of B-cell precursors.

We have raised a rabbit antiserum to p53 biochemically purified from methylcholanthrene-induced mouse sarcoma, Meth A (13). With this antiserum, immunofluorescence was reinvestigated using viable cells of Meth A and a murine embryonal carcinoma, F9. Our results are shown in Fig. 1. Clearly, fluorescence was detected on the cell surface as a granular staining on both the Meth A and the

FIG. 1. Reactions of rabbit anti p53 antiserum in indirect immunofluorescence tests, with **A:** Meth A sarcoma cells, **B:** 12-1a cells (pBR322/HSV-1tk/SV40-transformed F9 cells treated with retinoic acid) (17), and **C:** F9 cells.

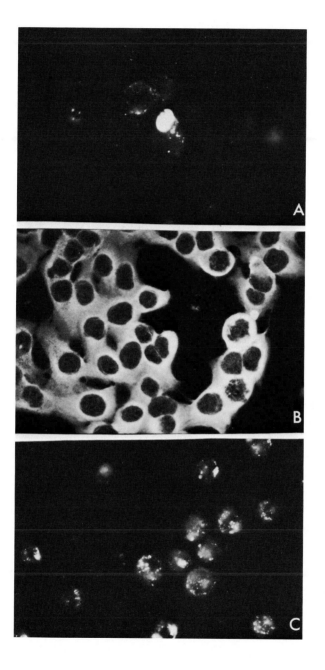

F9 cells. However, when these cells were fixed by methanol-acetone, an irregular cytoplasmic staining was obtained. A cloned cell line that was derived from F9, termed 12-1a, which contained one copy of the SV40 genome and expressed SV40 T antigen after treatment with retinoic acid, was also used for our immunofluorescence studies (Fig. 1). The fluorescence was demonstrable with the same distribution as T antigen. Results that were obtained from cellular fractionation experiments also have indicated that large amounts of both T antigen and p53 protein were present together in the nuclear fraction and, in a lesser amount, in the plasma membrane fraction (19).

At present it is well established that there are two patterns of distribution of intracellular p53. Most cells have an irregular cytoplasmic distribution. Cells that contain the SV40 T antigen display a marked shift of p53 to peri- and intranuclear locations. The surface expression of p53 is presently a more difficult problem; depending on the cell line examined and the reagents used, p53 may or may not be demonstrable. Although these results suggest that surface expression of p53 may represent an important differentiation antigen, purely technical questions must be resolved first. The distribution pattern of p53 in various components of the cell may prove to be very important. One obvious possibility is that p53 may be able to express its function(s) from different intracellular locations, and there might be a requirement of a membrane association for transformation. However, such relationships still remain to be characterized.

BIOCHEMICAL PROPERTIES OF p53

The p53 proteins have been detected in a variety of transformed cells of different species. To examine the structural relationships between these proteins, they have been analyzed by a variety of biochemical techniques. To determine whether p53 is a phosphoprotein, cells were labeled with $^{32}PO_4$ and immunoprecipitated with either conventional or monoclonal antibodies. In both the murine and human cells, ^{32}P-labeled p53 was immunoprecipitated from the lysates, clearly demonstrating that p53 is a phosphoprotein (5,11). Experiments designed to show whether p53 is a glycoprotein were not definitive: two different studies have been carried out and both indicated that p53 is not glycosylated. In the first experiment, a ^{35}S-methionine-labeled lysate of an Abelson-transformed mouse cell line (2M3/M) was precipitated with anti p53 antiserum and then treated with endo-βacetylglucosaminidase H. No change in the electrophoretic mobility of p53 was apparent after such treatment (11). In a second experiment, treatment of human cells during growth *in vitro* with tunicamycin, a specific inhibitor of glycosylation, also had no effect on the electrophoretic mobility of p53 (5). Despite these results, it is still possible to argue that carbohydrate moieties are present on p53; a definitive answer will be obtained by direct carbohydrate analysis of purified p53.

Comparison of p53 from different cell lines has been carried out using two-dimensional gel electrophoresis. With both murine and human p53, the most common pattern observed was a streak of multiple spots, with a major protein species of pI between 6.3 and 6.7, and a minor species with a pI around 7.2 (5,6). Differences in the isoelectric focusing patterns of p53 from different cell preparations have been noted, but their significance is unclear.

Fingerprinting analyses of p53 have also been carried out. Initial results have shown that tryptic digests of ^{35}S-methionine-labeled p53 from SV40-transformed mouse cells had no peptides in common with large T or small t antigens of SV40 (1,32). Further work has clearly established that tryptic peptide maps of p53 obtained from mouse cell lines transformed by SV40, polyoma virus, Moloney murine leukemia virus (M-MuLV), or Schmidt-Ruppin avian sarcoma virus (ASV), were very similar (11). Fingerprinting analyses of ^{35}S-labeled or ^{14}C-labeled p53 antigens obtained from four different murine methylcholanthrene-induced sarcomas also showed a high degree of similarity of their tryptic digests. Similar or identical peptide maps have been obtained from murine embryonal carcinoma cells, F9, BALB/c 3T12 cells, and an *in vitro* translation product of mRNA from SV40-transformed cells (21). The p53 proteins isolated from each of these sources had eight methionine-containing

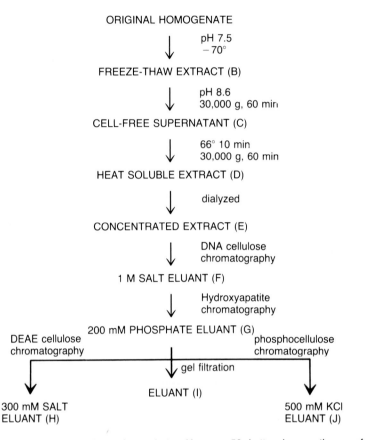

FIG. 2. Purification scheme for murine and human p53. *Letters in parentheses* refer to protein fractions separated by gel electrophoresis, and shown in Fig. 3.

peptides in common with the p53 protein obtained after *in vivo* labeling of SV40-transformed cells in culture. These results demonstrated the structural similarities of the p53 proteins derived from a variety of murine cells transformed by diverse agents. The p53 proteins immunoprecipitated from different human tumor cell lines have been examined by partial proteolytic cleavage, and the results have shown that the various p53 proteins are also very similar (5). A comparison of the p53 proteins from murine and human tissues using proteolytic cleavage has shown many similarities, although

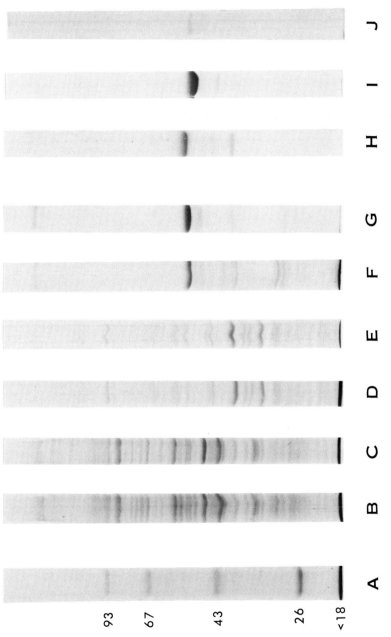
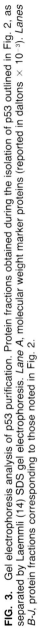

93

67

43

26

<18

A B C D E F G H I J

FIG. 3. Gel electrophoresis analysis of p53 purification. Protein fractions obtained during the isolation of p53 outlined in Fig. 2, as separated by Laemmli (14) SDS gel electrophoresis. *Lane A*, molecular weight marker proteins (reported in daltons $\times$ 10^{-3}). *Lanes B-J*, protein fractions corresponding to those noted in Fig. 2.

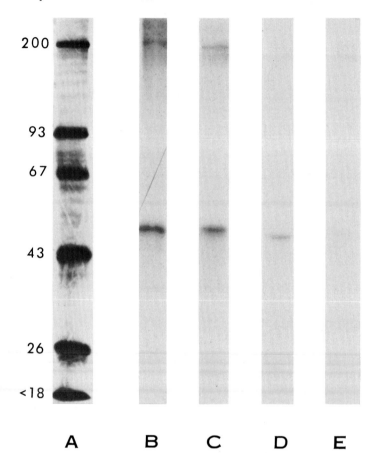

FIG. 4. Immunoprecipitation of purified p53. p53 was isolated as described in Fig. 2 and iodinated with Bolton and Hunter reagent. Immunoprecipitation assays were set up with monoclonal antisera, and the precipitated proteins were subsequently separated on 7.5% Laemmli SDS gels. *Lane A*, ^{14}C molecular weight standards (reported in daltons $\times$ 10^{-3}). *Lane B*, purified ^{125}I-p53. *Lanes C–E*, ^{125}I-p53 immunoprecipitated with: *Lane C*, anti p53 rat monoclonal RA3-2C2; *Lane D*, anti p53 mouse monoclonal 200-20; *Lane E*, control, mouse monoclonal Ly 2.2.

some differences were detectable (13). Further tryptic digest analysis of p53 proteins from rat or hamster cells has shown that these proteins are also closely related (31). Thus, to date there is no clear evidence indicating structural heterogeneity among the p53 proteins.

Another biochemical parameter of p53 that has been examined is its association with a kinase activity (12). Extracts of Meth A or 3T3 WT (an SV40-transformed 3T3 cell line), were allowed to react with a murine anti p53 monoclonal antibody, and the resulting immune complex was incubated with γ-^{32}P-ATP to assay for protein kinase activity. p53 was selectively autophosphorylated in immunoprecipitates of Meth A and 3T3 WT cells. This enzymatic activity was dependent on divalent cation concentration; the activity obtained with Mn^{2+} was at least fivefold higher than that with Mg^{2+}. This dependency resembles the one reported for pp60[src] kinase of avian sarcoma virus and the pl20 kinase of Abelson MuLV (29,34). Analysis of the amino acids of p53 that were phosphorylated showed that both serine and threonine were phosphorylated in the immune complex assay, but no phosphotyrosine was evident. These same amino acids have been reported to act as acceptors for the kinases associated with the transforming proteins of both SV40 and adenovirus *in vitro* (8,16).

Another characteristic of p53 that has been described is its ability to form complexes with the virus-coded large T antigen in murine cells transformed by SV40 (24). These complexes sediment with a molecular weight of between 600K to 1,000K; they are held together by noncovalent bonds and are located in the cell nucleus. The complexed form of large T antigen can be more readily phosphorylated than the free form. Formation of similar complexes have also been shown in extracts of SV40-infected, SV-1 African green monkey kidney cells (10). Both large T antigen and p53 phosphoproteins have been precipitated from lysates of infected CV-1 cells by antibodies specific for either component of the complex. An important observation was a significant increase in the amounts of ^{35}S-methionine and ^{32}P-phosphate incorporated into the p53 protein on infection of CV-1 cells with SV40. This modification of the rates of synthesis and phosphorylation of the p53 protein may be essential for some stage of the SV40 life cycle. Further work recently published has demonstrated the direct interaction of highly purified T antigen (D2 T antigen or SV80 T antigen) with p53 in lysates from a variety of murine cell lines (23). Further study should allow a more accurate assessment of whether the binding of p53 affects the biochemical activity of T antigen, and thus might modify its biological functions.

PURIFICATION OF p53 AND PARTIAL STRUCTURE

Purification of p53 has been attempted from Meth A murine sarcoma, a TA3 murine mammary carcinoma, and two human cell lines, Raji and Mamalwa, derived from Burkitt's lymphomas. The purification method essentially is the one outlined by Luka et al. (20) with modifications as described in Fig. 2. The procedure takes advantage of the two basic facts that the p53 proteins are heat-stable and that they have DNA-binding capacity. To date, we have successfully performed the purification scheme several times, with an average recovery of about 25% and an increase in the specific activity of p53 of about 400 times. We have raised a rabbit antiserum to purified p53 and have developed a highly specific and sensitive radioimmunoassay that has been used to follow the purification. The data we have obtained thus far indicate that p53 is present in the original cellular homogenate at an initial concentration of approximately 0.1%.

It should be noted that p53 is extremely susceptible to proteolysis, and great care must be taken to maintain low temperature and adequate concentrations of protease inhibitors throughout the purification. In addition, p53 readily forms a tetramer, and this in turn appears to polymerize further to form extremely high molecular weight aggregates. The purification scheme is summarized as follows:

The ascites cells are washed, then frozen at $-70°$ C. The following day, the cells are thawed rapidly while raising the pH of the extraction buffer from 7.5 to 8.6. The solubilized proteins are separated by centrifugation, then subjected to heat extraction at $65°$ C for 10 min. After rapid chilling, the p53 is recovered from the precipitable proteins by centrifugation and further purified by calf thymus DNA-cellulose chromatography. After eluting the unbound proteins from the column, p53 is eluted with an increase in the salt concentration. Finally, a hydroxyapatite purification step is performed, separating unbound proteins from the bound p53 by an increase in phosphate concentration. Determination of p53 purity by analytical gel electrophoresis and by radioimmunoassay indicate that p53 is about 50% pure through the hydroxyapatite step; the contaminants remaining are one high molecular weight species, and several low molecular weight ones. Since p53 is a protein that aggregates readily, further purification efforts have been relatively difficult. We have succeeded in obtaining small quantities of pure p53 by DEAE-Sephadex chromatography, by phosphocellulose chromatography, and by conventional gel filtration, but yields of less than 10% have been obtained. The protein banding patterns throughout the purification scheme are shown in Fig. 3.

The purified p53 shows essentially one band on SDS-polyacrylamide gel electrophoresis, with only trace amounts of bands corresponding to lower molecular weight contaminants. Analysis of purified fractions by high pressure liquid chromatography also showed a single protein peak. To ensure that the p53 isolated by this purification scheme was identical to the immunoprecipitable p53, immunoprecipitation assays were carried out with iodinated purified p53 and two different monoclonal antibodies to p53. Analysis of the resulting immunoprecipitates (shown in Fig. 4) confirm that these antibodies did recognize the purified p53.

Partial structural analysis of p53 has been performed on the purified p53 preparations obtained from the murine and human cell lines (13). These proteins are very similar in amino acid composition and have closely related peptide maps. The amino acid sequences of the first 20 residues of p53 from murine and human sources were identical; no similarities were found with the large T antigen from SV40, the middle T antigen of polyoma virus, or the immunoglobulin heavy chains.

CONCLUSION

We have summarized the known characteristics of p53 in the preceding text; these are outlined in Table 2. It has become obvious

TABLE 2. *Summary of human and murine p53 characteristics*

Expressed at elevated levels in all transformed cells
Not detectable in slowly dividing or static cells
Intracellularly located primarily within the nucleus, but may be distributed in the cytoplasm or on the plasma membrane under certain conditions
Monomer M_R is 53,000 daltons
Isoelectric point is 6.3 to 6.7
Readily polymerizes to form tetramer, and will aggregate to form higher molecular weight complexes
Associates specifically with large T antigen if available
Can be phosphorylated
Appears not to be glycosylated
Heat stable and soluble
Binds tightly to DNA
Displays Mn^{2+} dependent kinase activity
Highly conserved in all species

that p53 from a variety of different transformed cells of various species is a highly conserved protein. The functional role of p53 still remains undefined. However, regulation of cell division is perhaps the most plausible possibility. In this regard, one important observation is that p53 cannot be detected in nondividing lymphocytes, but its synthesis, and/or expression, is induced when cells enter the division cycle in response to Con A stimulation (25). To date, p53 is the only detectable protein that is newly expressed and it can be detected within 4 hr following Con A stimulation. This strongly suggests that p53 may be involved in the commitment of cells to enter the division cycle. When mRNA synthesis is reversibly blocked by α-amanitin, the induction of p53 is also blocked. All these data indicate that the expression of p53 is tightly controlled at the level of p53 gene transcription.

In malignant cells, several types of genetic or epigenetic events could lead to loss of this control over cell division; the elevated rate of synthesis of p53 may account for the loss of control of division. An alternative possibility is that the elevated level of p53 is secondary to cellular transformation. The binding of p53 by large T antigen in SV40-transformed cells, and possibly by transforming proteins of other DNA and RNA viruses, may disrupt the cellular balance of p53 levels, and result in persistently high concentrations of functional p53. This would be consistent with the recent observation that the level of translatable p53 mRNA from 3T3, and from SV40-transformed 3T3 cells, were roughly equivalent (27). Another observation consistent with the above possibility is that p53 antigens are highly conserved proteins since they have to interact with SV40 large T antigen, and other structures from very different types of cells.

A further consideration that should be entertained is the observation that transforming proteins act as a kinase. If the products of viral transforming genes are in fact kinases, then the p53 protein may well serve as a specific phosphoacceptor. Such macromolecular interaction may represent one mechanism of action of the viral transforming protein producing the cellular changes associated with transformation.

ACKNOWLEDGMENTS

The authors wish to express their thanks to Dr. Kenichi Tanaka for his help with the immunofluorescence study, to Dr. Carlo Croce for the F9, 12-1, and 12-1a cells, and to Ms. Victoria Armstrong for her expertise in preparing the manuscript.

REFERENCES

1. Chang, C., Simmons, D. T., Martin, M. A., and Mora, P. T. (1979): Identification and partial characterization of new species of SV40 specific antigens from SV40 transformed mouse embryo cell lines. *J. Virol.*, 31:463–471.
2. Coffman, R. L., and Weissman, I. L. (1981): A monoclonal antibody which recognizes B cells and B cell precursors in mice. *J. Exp. Med.*, 153:269–279.
3. Collett, M. S., Brugge, J. S., and Erikson, R. L. (1978): Characterization of a normal avian cell protein related to the avian sarcoma virus transforming gene product. *Cell*, 15:1363–1369.
4. Collett, M. S., and Erikson, R. L. (1978): Protein kinase activity associated with the avian sarcoma virus src gene product. *Proc. Natl. Acad. Sci. USA*, 75:2021–2024.
5. Crawford, L. V., Pim, D. C., Gurney, E. G., Goodfellow, P., and Taylor-Papadimitriou, J. (1981): Detection of a common feature in several human tumor cell lines: A 53,000-dalton protein. *Proc. Natl. Acad. Sci. USA*, 78:41–45.

6. DeLeo, A. B., Jay, G., Appella, E., DuBois, G. C., Law, L. W., and Old, L. J. (1979): Detection of a transformation-related antigen in chemically induced sarcomas and other transformed cells of the mouse. *Proc. Natl. Acad. Sci. USA*, 76:2420–2424.

7. Dippold, W. G., Jay, G., DeLeo, A. B., Khoury, G., and Old, L. J. (1981): P53 transformation-related protein: Detection by monoclonal antibody in mouse and human cells. *Proc. Natl. Acad. Sci. USA*, 78:1695–1699.

8. Griffin, J. D., Spangler, G., and Livingston, D. M. (1979): Protein kinase activity associated with simian virus 40 T antigen. *Proc. Natl. Acad. Sci. USA*, 76:2610–2614.

9. Gurney, E. G., Harrison, R. O., and Fenno, J. (1980): Monoclonal antibodies against Simian virus 40 T antigens: Evidence for distinct subclasses of large T antigen and for similarities among nonviral T antigens. *J. Virol.*, 34:752–763.

10. Harlow, E., Pim, D. C., and Crawford, L. V. (1981): Complex of simian virus 40 large T antigen and host 53,000 molecular weight protein in monkey cells. *J. Virol.*, 37:564–573.

11. Jay, G., DeLeo, A. B., Appella, E., DuBois, G. C., Law, L. W., Khoury, G., and Old, L. J. (1980): A common transformation-related protein in murine sarcomas and leukemias. *Cold Spring Harbor Symp. Quant. Biol.*, 44:659–664.

12. Jay, G., Khoury, G., DeLeo, A. B., Dippold, W. G., and Old, L. J. (1981): P53 transformation-related protein: Detection of an associated phosphotransferase activity. *Proc. Natl. Acad. Sci. USA*, 78:2932–2936.

13. Jornvall, H., Luka, J., Klein, G., and Appella, E. (1982): A 53K protein common to chemically and virally transformed cells shows extensive sequence similarities between species. *Proc. Natl. Acad. Sci. USA*, 79:287–291.

14. Laemmli, U. K. (1970): Cleavage of structural proteins during the assembly of the head of bacteriophage T4. *Nature*, 227:680–685.

15. Lane, D. P., and Crawford, L. V. (1979): T antigen is bound to a host protein in SV40 transformed cells. *Nature*, 278:261–263.

16. Lassam, N. J., Bayley, S. T., Graham, F. L., and Branton, P. E. (1979): Immunoprecipitation of protein kinase activity from adenovirus 5-infected cells using antiserum directed against tumor antigens. *Nature*, 277:241–243.

17. Linnenbach, A., Huebner, K., and Croce, C. M. (1980): DNA-transformed murine teratocarcinoma cells: Regulation of expression of simian virus 40 tumor antigen in stem versus differentiated cells. *Proc. Natl. Acad. Sci. USA*, 77:4875–4879.

18. Linzer, D. I. H., and Levine, A. J. (1979): Characterization of a 54K dalton cellular SV40 tumor antigen present in SV40-transformed cells and uninfected embryonal carcinoma cells. *Cell*, 17:43–52.

19. Luborsky, S. W., and Chandrasekaran, K. (1980): Subcellular distribution of Simian virus 40 T antigen species in various cell lines: The 56K protein. *Int. J. Cancer*, 25:517–527.

20. Luka, J., Jornvall, H., and Klein, G. (1980): Purification and biochemical characterization of the Epstein-Barr virus-determined nuclear antigen and an associated protein with a 53,000 dalton subunit. *J. Virol.*, 35:592–602.
21. Maltzman, W., Oren, M., and Levine, A. J. (1981): The structural relationships between 54,000-molecular weight cellular tumor antigens detected in viral- and non-viral transformed cells. *Virology*, 112:145–156.
22. Martin, R. G. (1981): The transformation of cell growth and transmogrification of DNA synthesis by simian virus 40. *Adv. Cancer Res.*, 34:1–68.
23. McCormick, F., Clark, R., Harlow, E., and Tijan, R. (1981): SV40 T antigen binds specifically to a cellular 53K protein *in vitro*. *Nature*, 292:63–65.
24. McCormick, F., and Harlow, E. (1980): Association of a murine 53,000 dalton phosphoprotein with simian virus 40 large T antigen in transformed cells. *J. Virol.*, 34:213–224.
25. Milner, J., and Milner, S. (1981): SV40-53K antigen: A possible role for 53K in normal cells. *Virology*, 112:785–788.
26. Oppermann, H., Levinson, A. D., Varmus, H. E., Levintow, L., and Bishop, J. M. (1979): Uninfected vertebrate cells contain a protein that is closely related to the product of the avian sarcoma virus transforming gene (src). *Proc. Natl. Acad. Sci. USA*, 76:1804–1808.
27. Oren, M., Maltzman, W., and Levine, A. J. (1981): Post-translational regulation of the 54K cellular tumor antigen in normal and transformed cells. *Mol. Cell. Biol.*, 1:101–110.
28. Purchio, A. F., Erikson, E., and Erikson, R. L. (1977): Translation of 35S and of subgenomic regions of avian sarcoma virus RNA. *Proc. Natl. Acad. Sci. USA*, 74:4661–4665.
29. Richert, N. D., Davies, P. J. A., Jay, G., and Pastan, I. H. (1979): Characterization of an immune complex kinase in immunoprecipitates of avian sarcoma virus-transformed fibroblasts. *J. Virol.*, 31:695–706.
30. Rotter, V., Witte, O. N., Coffman, R., and Baltimore, D. (1980): Abelson murine leukemia virus-induced tumors elicit antibodies against a host cell protein, P50. *J. Virol.*, 36:547–555.
31. Simmons, D. T., Martin, M. A., Mora, P. T., and Chang, C. (1980): Relationship among Tau antigens isolated from various lines of Simian virus 40-transformed cells. *J. Virol.*, 34:650–657.
32. Smith, A. E., Smith, R., and Paucha, E. (1979): Characterization of different tumor antigens present in cells transformed by Simian virus 40. *Cell*, 18:335–346.
33. Weil, R. (1978): Viral tumor antigens. A novel type of mammalian regulator protein. *Biochim. Biophys. Acta*, 516:301–388.
34. Witte, O. N., Dasgupta, A., and Baltimore, D. (1980): Abelson murine leukaemia virus protein is phosphorylated *in vitro* to form phosphotyrosine. *Nature*, 283:826–831.
35. Witte, O. N., Rosenberg, N. E., and Baltimore, D. (1979): A normal cell protein cross-reactive to the major Abelson murine leukaemia virus gene product. *Nature*, 281:396–398.

Advances in Viral Oncology, Volume 2, edited by
George Klein. Raven Press, New York © 1982.

The DNA-Binding Protein p53 in Epstein-Barr Virus Transformed Cells
Properties of This Protein, Other p53 Forms, and the Epstein-Barr Virus Nuclear Antigen

*Janos Luka and **Hans Jörnvall

*Departments of *Tumor Biology and **Chemistry I, Karolinska Institutet,
S-104 01 Stockholm, Sweden*

Among the different types of tumor-associated antigens, a soluble protein (p53) with polypeptides of approximately 53,000 in molecular weight has been detected in many transformed cells. One such protein is associated with the large viral T-antigen in SV 40 transformed cells (2,8,21,23). A p53 also occurs in chemically induced mouse sarcomas (3) and in Epstein-Barr virus transformed B-cell lines, from which p53 has been purified by using a DNA binding step (25). One important question concerns the relationship between these (and other) p53 forms. It should be noted that SV 40 and Epstein-Barr virus are highly different in type. The Epstein-Barr virus is much larger and interacts with cells in a strategically different way. Already these two viral transformations therefore illustrate the question of p53 relationships, although p53s are known to be of host-cell origin. A second question is if p53s indicate a common transformation mechanism, especially since such proteins appear to link chemically- and virally-induced transformations, associate with T-antigens, and bind to DNA.

In this review, we shall summarize our results on p53 and an associated protein in the Epstein-Barr virus system. With reference to the question of relationships among different p53 forms, we shall also discuss structural investigations of some p53 molecules of different origin.

TRANSFORMATION BY EPSTEIN-BARR VIRUS

The Epstein-Barr Virus

Epstein-Barr virus was demonstrated by Epstein et al. (4), in a cell line derived from an African Burkitt lymphoma. The virus was later shown to be regularly associated with this type of tumor, with a type of nasopharyngeal carcinoma, and with infectious mononucleosis (12,36). Studies on the molecular biology of the virus have suffered from a lack of a known lytic system for virus production. Only a low percentage of the cells in some transformed cell lines express viral antigens associated with the lytic cycle and produce small amounts of virus. Although several agents increase the number of cells that express early and late virus antigens (6,9,10,26,41), they increase virus production only slightly.

Two infectious virus prototypes are widely used. One, the B95-8 substrain, is of mononucleosis origin and carried in a marmoset-derived B-lymphocyte line (30). The other, the P3HR-1 substrain, is of tumor origin and produced by a human Burkitt lymphoma line (15). Infection of human B-lymphocytes with the B95-8 virus is nonproductive and results in transformation or immortalization *in vitro*. The P3HR-1 strain cannot transform lymphocytes *in vitro* but can induce an abortive virus cycle by superinfection of Epstein-Barr virus-genome positive cells (13,14). Cell lines that have been used as starting material for the protein purifications reviewed here are the Burkitt lymphoma lines Raji and Namalva, which carry the Epstein-Barr virus genome but are virus nonproducers. The Epstein-Barr virus negative American Burkitt lymphoma line Ramos has also been used as a source for p53 purification.

Epstein-Barr virus DNA has a molecular weight of 100×10^6, and the genome has been partly characterized by mapping with restriction enzymes (7,11). The P3HR-1 virus DNA is highly similar to the B95-8 virus DNA, but it contains a deletion in the EcoRI A fragment. The Epstein-Barr virus-genome in transformed cells is present in multiple copies. Most of these exist as free plasmids in the form of covalently closed circles (22), but some copies may also be integrated.

Epstein-Barr Virus-Determined Nuclear Antigen

Epstein-Barr virus-associated antigens are usually detected with human sera containing antibodies to different combinations of the virus-associated proteins. Two antigens, Epstein-Barr virus-determined nuclear antigen (EBNA) (33) and the lymphocyte-detected membrane antigen LYDMA (38), are present in transformed cells, whereas the early antigen (EA) complex, membrane antigen (MA), and virus capsid antigen (VCA) are associated with the lytic cycle (18).

The Epstein-Barr virus-determined nuclear antigen was first demonstrated by Reedman and Klein 1973 (33), using the sensitive anticomplement immunofluorescence assay. Virus-genome positive cells showed a fine granular nuclear fluorescence, whereas none of the virus-genome negative cells was stained by antibodies from seropositive individuals. Immunofluorescence studies showed that EBNA is associated with metaphase chromosomes (31,33). A direct linear relationship appears to exist between the number of virus DNA copies per cell as determined by molecular hybridization and the amount of EBNA per nucleus (5,35).

All virus-genome positive cell lines have also been reported to express a heat-stable soluble (S) complement-fixing antigen (34,43). Available data suggest that the S-antigen and EBNA are identical (20). Thus, the S-antigen binds to DNA (1,28) and to metaphase chromosomes (31), and its isoelectric point (29) and molecular weight are similar to partially purified EBNA from chromatin.

IDENTIFICATION AND PURIFICATION OF EBNA

In initial attempts to isolate EBNA, detergent treatments were used but with limited success. The intranuclear localization of EBNA and its binding to metaphase chromosomes led to the use of DNA-cellulose chromatography in EBNA purifications (1,28). It was applied as the first step in a four-step procedure to purify the antigen (27). The heat stability of EBNA was utilized in a subsequent purification scheme, producing apparently homogeneous 48K-EBNA polypeptide (25). Analysis of this preparation showed that EBNA was a hydrophilic protein, distinct from p53 but with a similar overall composition (25).

Further studies have shown that EBNA prepared by this method, based on heat treatment and DNA-cellulose chromatography, is not always recovered as a homogeneous 48K polypeptide. Thus, sequence analysis of the preparation revealed the presence of different N-terminal sequences (17), and similar purifications in other laboratories produced EBNA-active preparations with polypeptides of higher molecular weight (65K-81K) (37).

All these observations reveal that the native polypeptide size and properties of EBNA are not fully established. It is possible that the different sizes reflect proteolysis products from a larger polypeptide and that the 48K form is the smallest fragment with EBNA activity. Proteolytic processing would be compatible with the apparent heterogeneity of the 48K-EBNA preparation (17) and with the presence of different EBNA products in different cells (37). However, this possibility remains to be investigated, and the relationship between the different EBNA forms is not yet known. It is clear, however, that the antigenic activity of EBNA as judged by fluorescence staining is separately associated with the various polypeptide sizes reported, as shown in Fig. 1. The original observation on the composition of the 48K component and its nonidentity with p53 is therefore still valid.

IDENTIFICATION AND PURIFICATION OF p53

Characterization of the Protein from Different Sources

In immunoprecipitation experiments, antiEBNA positive sera precipitate two polypeptides from ^{14}C-labeled Epstein-Barr virus-ge-

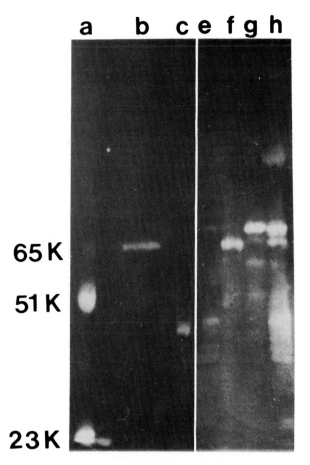

FIG. 1. Fluorescence immunoelectrophoresis of EBNA from different purifications. (a) FITC-labeled IgG marker, (b) 65K-EBNA from Raji cells, (c) 48K-EBNA from Raji cells, (e) staphylococcal protease-treated 70K-EBNA from P3HR-1 cells, (f) 65K-EBNA from Raji cells, (g) 70K-EBNA from P3HR-1 cells, (h) degradation products from 70K-EBNA in TPA + butyrate-induced P3HR-1 cells.

nome positive cells (25). Controls show that no polypeptides are precipitated from Epstein-Barr virus negative cells by these sera, or from Raji cells by antiEBNA negative sera (Fig. 2). On SDS-poly-acrylamide gel electrophoresis, the molecular weights of the im-munoprecipitated polypeptides are approximately 48,000,

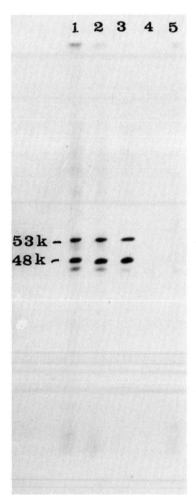

FIG. 2. Immunoprecipitation followed by SDS-polyacrylamide gel electrophoresis of ^{14}C-labeled 48K-EBNA and p53 from Raji cells. Lanes 1,2,3: three different antiEBNA positive sera; lanes 4,5: two different antiEBNA negative sera.

corresponding to 48K-EBNA, and 53,000, corresponding to p53. In addition, studies of differently pretreated extracts suggest that the 53K polypeptide may also give rise to chains of lower molecular weights, probably as a result of proteolysis. This prompts the use of protease inhibitors and quick steps in p53 purification (17). The coprecipitation of p53 and the 48K form of EBNA by antiEBNA antibodies (Fig. 2) may suggest that EBNA (at least the 48K poly-peptide form) is bound to p53. This evidence obtained in the Epstein-Barr virus system closely resembles the findings that were inter-preted to indicate an association between a p53 and the SV 40 large T-antigen (21).

A p53 protein has been purified from Raji cells, by using the same scheme as for the EBNA preparation (25). This is shown in Fig. 3. In the initial purification steps, the 48K-EBNA and p53 copurify. The DNA-cellulose chromatography step gives a highly effective purification. After this step, essentially only three major polypeptide types were detected by electrophoresis: p53, 48K-EBNA, and the high-mobility group (HMG) proteins. These three types of protein are separated on hydroxyapatite chromatography. In the presence of 200 mM NaCl, p53 elutes first with 50 mM phosphate, followed by EBNA with 180 mM phosphate, and finally HMG with 400 mM phosphate.

With the purification scheme in Fig. 3, p53 can also be prepared from Epstein-Barr virus-genome negative lymphoma cell lines (Ra-mos). The p53 proteins are highly similar from Epstein-Barr virus negative (Ramos) and positive (Raji) cells (25). Together with the successful purification of p53 from still other cells (17), this proves that the protein is of cellular origin, in contrast to EBNA that can be obtained only from Epstein-Barr virus-genome carrying cells. By using the method in Fig. 3, p53 has been demonstrated by subsequent gel electrophoresis in several differently transformed cells of human and mouse origin. As listed in Table 1, they include the methyl-cholanthrene-induced sarcoma Meth-A, SV 40 transformed rat fi-broblasts, and a mouse mammary carcinoma line (17).

This method does not allow proper quantitation, but the amount of p53 estimated from ^{14}C-labeled cells appears to vary between different cell lines. The largest amounts were recovered from Ep-stein-Barr virus transformed cells and from the Meth-A sarcoma. It is estimated to be present in smaller amounts in the Epstein-Barr virus-genome negative lymphoma lines, but Epstein-Barr virus con-

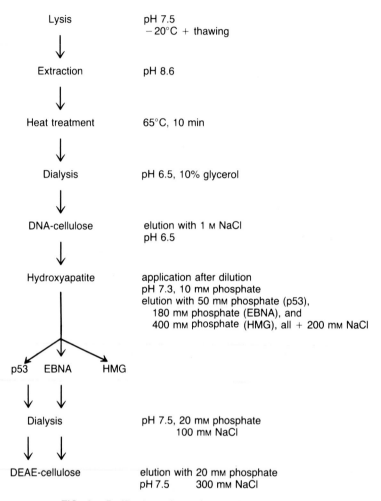

FIG. 3. Purification scheme for p53, EBNA, and HMG proteins.

version of them (Ramos to AW-Ramos) by superinfection with the P3HR-1 substrain appeared to increase their content of p53 (19). The protein was not detectable with this method in normal or mitogen-stimulated B-lymphocytes, and it was present in only very small amounts in T-cell lines derived from acute lymphatic leukemia (19).

TABLE 1. *Cells from which DNA-binding p53 has been detected by SDS-polyacrylamide gel electrophoresis after the DNA-cellulose chromatography step of the purification*

Cells	Species	Origin
Raji	Human	Burkitt lymphoma
Namalva	Human	Burkitt lymphoma
Ramos	Human	American Burkitt lymphoma
Bjab	Human	Burkitt lymphoma
Meth-A	Mouse	Methylcholanthrene induced carcinoma
TA-3	Mouse	Mouse mammary carcinoma
SV 40 Rat-1	Rat	SV 40 transformed fibroblast
Rat-1 wtz	Rat	Polyoma transformed fibroblast
Rat-1 wty	Rat	Polyoma transformed fibroblast

We have also found that two different forms of p53 may occur in one cell. These forms can be separated by DEAE-Sephadex chromatography and can also be resolved on gel electrophoresis in acidic urea. It appears that Epstein-Barr virus positive cell lines contain both forms, whereas preliminary studies suggest that virus negative cell lines have only one form (25). The two forms have been called $p53_c$ and $p53_u$ (for *c*ommon to both types of cells, and *u*nique to virus positive cells). The exact relationship between these two forms is unknown, but the structural differences are small and may correspond to single modifications.

Immunological and Functional Studies

As mentioned above, p53 prepared from human cells does not express EBNA activity in the immunological tests performed. However, it increases the apparent titer of 48K-EBNA activity in the complement fixation test and in the acid-fixed nuclear binding assay (25). An *in vitro* association between p53 and 48K-EBNA has also been suggested because incubation of a mixture of the purified ^{14}C-labeled proteins with antiEBNA positive sera brings down both proteins in an apparently equimolar ratio (25). Since two p53 forms occur (25), it may be noticed that the complex was found independently of whether the p53 used was derived from Epstein-Barr virus positive or negative human cell lines (25).

Tests with 48K-EBNA for inhibition of leukocyte migration suggest a similar association. In contrast to crude extracts of Epstein-Barr virus-carrying cells or to native EBNA extracts, p53 alone had no effect on the leukocyte migration from seropositive individuals. Purified 48K-EBNA was strongly inhibitory on leukocytes from seropositive donors at a concentration of 10 μg/ml, but it had no significant effect at 5 μg/ml. The mixture of 48K-EBNA and p53 was already strongly inhibitory at a concentration of 5 μg/ml (39,40).

Preliminary experiments with rabbit sera directed against 48K-EBNA, p53, and HMG proteins demonstrated a specific reaction with human p53 in a micro-ELISA assay (Sternås et al., *in preparation*). This technique also showed a weak immunological cross-reaction with p53 of murine origin. However, in the leukocyte migration assay, the mouse p53 did not enhance the effect of the 48K-EBNA (40), in contrast to the human p53 preparation. This is interesting because mouse lymphocytes respond to artificial Epstein-Barr virus injection by entering into the lytic cycle with little or no EBNA production. It is tempting to speculate that the different courses of events—EBNA synthesis with transformation in the human lymphocyte versus lytic infection with little or no EBNA in the mouse lymphocyte—may be related to the differences in the interaction between EBNA and p53 of the two species. This hypothesis is similar to the suggestion regarding the role of T-antigen binding to p53 in the SV 40 system (G. Klein, *this volume*), although transformation does not always appear to be directly correlated with the presence of the T-antigen–p53 complex (A. J. Levine, *this volume*).

Microinjection of purified 48K-EBNA into 3T3 fibroblasts stimulates cellular DNA synthesis (19). It remains to be seen whether p53 or 48K-EBNA is responsible for the mitogenic effect.

FIG. 4. Analysis of bound 48K-EBNA, p53, and HMG proteins to SV 40 DNA on sucrose gradient. *(a)* Ramos (EBNA negative) DNA-cellulose purified p53 and HMG; *(b)* individually purified Raji 48K-EBNA, p53, and HMG; *(c)* DNA-cellulose purified Raji 48K-EBNA, p53, and HMG.

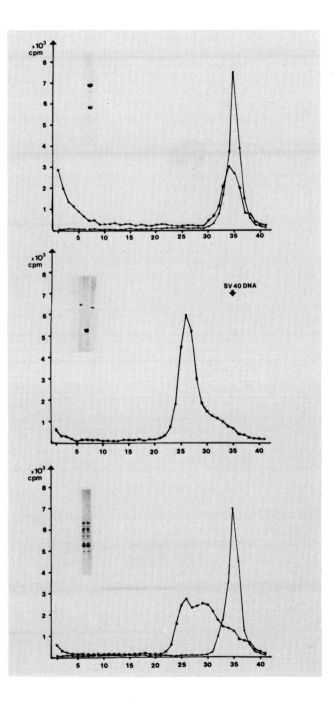

In DNA binding studies, mixtures of 48K-EBNA, p53, and HMG were found to bind to SV 40 DNA form I. Analysis on a sucrose gradient showed that the complexed DNA sediments as a 60 S component. Further analysis with purified components suggested that all three proteins are probably needed for this effect (Fig. 4). At high protein concentrations, the DNA was precipitated. The effect on SV 40 DNA was independent of whether the p53 used was derived from Epstein-Barr virus positive or negative cells (J. Luka and B. Kallin, *unpublished results*).

Structural Studies

The Quaternary Structure

Sedimentation values of p53 have been determined in both the presence and absence of EBNA (25). The p53 from virus-genome positive or negative cell lines has a sedimentation coefficient of approximately 8.2 S. On Sephacryl S-300 chromatography, this corresponds to a molecular weight of approximately 200,000 for globular proteins, which would suggest that tetrameric structures are major constituents. The complex between 48K-EBNA and p53 has only a slightly different sedimentation coefficient of approximately 8.6 S. A complex formation in this aggregate is again supported by immunoprecipitation, which brings down both 48K-EBNA and p53. The 48K-EBNA alone also has a similar sedimentation coefficient, approximately 8.4 S. However, small amounts of proteins in all these preparations also sediment with coefficients up to 19 S, suggesting some aggregation. Although immunoprecipitation indicates a roughly equimolar ratio in the complex, the sedimentation studies do not show this, and the quaternary structures of all these molecules, p53, 48K-EBNA, and the complex, are not finally established. In the meantime, the sedimentation studies appear to suggest a predominant role of tetramers in all the protein forms.

The Primary Structure

The primary structure of p53 has been studied after purification from two human cell lines (Raji and Namalva) and from two murine cell lines (methylcholanthrene-induced Meth-A and TA-3 mammary carcinoma). Peptide mappings, utilizing CNBr or staphylococcal glutamic acid-specific protease, reveal great similarities. With the protease, three distinct polypeptides were obtained in all cases (Fig. 5), and with CNBr all proteins gave one large fragment at approximately 24 K. The two murine p53 forms are almost identical. The same is true for the two human forms, whereas the species appear

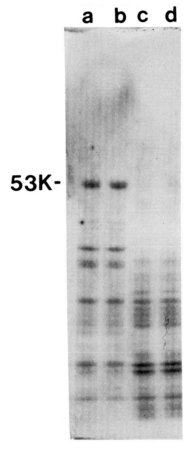

FIG. 5. SDS-polyacrylamide gel electrophoresis of four p53 proteins (a, Raji; b, Namalva; c, TA-3; d, Meth-A) after treatment with staphylococcal protease.

to differ in a few fragments (roughly 4 of 20 in the two types of digest) as judged by gel electrophoresis patterns.

The total compositions of all p53 preparations are highly similar (17,25). The composition is shown in Table 2 and compared with the 48K-EBNA composition (25). The cysteine content is low, and the whole p53 appears to be polar with an excess of dicarboxylic or amidated residues and glycine and with a low content of branched-chain or aromatic hydrophobic residues.

The N-terminal structures of the four p53 polypeptides have been analyzed (17), with identical results for the first 20 residues in all cases. This is shown in Table 3, revealing a largely polar structure, with a cysteine/half-cystine in position 10 and with a proline as the N-terminus.

TABLE 2. *Amino acid compositions of p53 preparations and 48K-EBNA[a]*

Amino acid	p53 from TA-3	48K-EBNA from Raji
Cys	0.9	
Asx	11.2	10.0
Thr	3.1	6.2
Ser	7.1	7.5
Glx	14.7	16.2
Pro	5.8	5.4
Gly	15.9	8.0
Ala	7.0	9.3
Val	4.5	5.7
Met	1.2	1.9
Ile	2.5	3.0
Leu	4.6	6.7
Tyr	0.9	1.7
Phe	3.4	2.8
Lys	8.2	9.2
His	2.3	1.4
Arg	6.8	5.1

[a]Values are given in mole percent, excluding tryptophan, and including cysteine/half-cystine only in TA-3. Within the mean standard deviation (0.6), different p53 preparations (Raji, Namalva, Meth-A, TA-3) showed largely similar values.

TABLE 3. *The N-terminal amino acid sequence of p53 preparations from human lymphoma lines (Raji, Namalva) and from mouse sarcoma (Meth-A) and mammary carcinoma (TA-3)*

Position	1		5				10				15					20
Sequence	Pro-Gly-His-Leu-Gln-Glu-Gly-Phe-Gly-Cys-Val-Val-Thr-Asn-Arg-Phe-Asp-Gln-Leu-Phe

Data from ref. 17.

The N-terminal structure has also been screened against several proteins with possibly related functions or structures (17). No significant homologies were detected, indicating that the characterized p53 structures appear to represent a unique type of polar, cellular, DNA-binding protein. The identical N-terminal structures, the similar peptide maps, and the closely related total compositions further show that p53 is a protein with an evolutionarily conserved structure. This indicates that it may have corresponding and important functions in mouse and human.

SUMMARY AND CONCLUSIONS

A cellular protein, p53, is emerging as a transformation-associated component in many animal and human tumors, as judged by the reports of such a protein in various systems (G. Klein, *this volume*). The question of whether high-level expression of this protein is essential for the maintenance of transformation in the cells where it occurs is of considerable importance.

In the SV 40 system, p53 complexes with the large T-antigen. As suggested by Levine *(this volume)*, the ability of large T-antigen to stabilize p53 may be an important part in the role played by large T in SV 40-induced transformation. This argument is strengthened by the finding that the Epstein-Barr virus-specified 48K-EBNA also appears to be associated with a p53 in a complex that may be similar in nature to the p53–large T complex in SV 40 transformed cells.

The EBNA-associated p53 has been purified from Epstein-Barr virus transformed human B-cell lines. The same protein was also found in Epstein-Barr virus negative B-lymphoma lines. Rabbit sera containing antibodies against human p53 showed a low cross-reactivity with murine p53 from nonvirally but methylcholanthrene-transformed sarcomas (Luka et al., *in preparation*). Furthermore, peptide mappings, amino acid compositions, and N-terminal sequence analyses clearly show that p53s from this sarcoma and from Epstein-Barr virus transformed B-cells are the same type of protein (17). Because other studies suggest an immunological cross-reactivity between p53 of SV 40 transformed cell lines and p53 of Meth-A sarcomas (3), it also appears likely that all these reports concern a common type of an important transformation-related p53 polypeptide.

The Epstein-Barr virus-carrying human host forms antibodies against the 48K subcomponent of EBNA, but an antibody response has not been detected against p53. The Epstein-Barr virus-specific leukocyte migration assay, designed to detect cell-mediated immunity of the human host to various Epstein-Barr virus antigens (40), gave similar results, showing sensitization to 48K-EBNA but not to p53 in Epstein-Barr virus seropositive individuals. However, addition of p53 to subliminal amounts of 48K-EBNA considerably enhanced the activity of the latter, as reflected by its immunological interaction with the sensitized lymphocytes in the inhibition tests of leukocyte migration. Human but not murine p53 appeared to act in this way. It is therefore conceivable that human p53 forms complexes with 48K-EBNA that are not formed by murine p53. If confirmed by direct biochemical studies, this finding may be relevant for understanding the role played by EBNA in transformation. Whereas human lymphocytes respond to Epstein-Barr virus infection with EBNA synthesis and immortalization, but essentially no lytic viral cycle, the artificial introduction of the virus into murine lymphocytes causes lytic infection (42). It is intriguing to speculate that this difference may relate to the ability of 48K-EBNA to complex with human but not with murine p53. Similar arguments apply to the role of p53–T-antigen complexes in SV 40 or adenovirus transformed cells (A. J. Levine, *this volume*).

The biological activity of p53 remains to be established. Phosphorylation mechanisms are particularly important to explore. A kinase activity appears associated with at least one p53 (16). The availability of pure p53 and the partial structural characterization of a few of these forms (17) open the way for comparisons with additional p53s and for further studies of the roles of p53 in transformation processes.

REFERENCES

1. Baron, D., and Strominger, J. L. (1978): *J. Biol. Chem.*, 253:2875–2881.
2. Crawford, L. V., Pim, D. C., Gurney, E. G., Goodfellow, P., and Taylor-Papadimitriou, J. (1981): *Proc. Natl. Acad. Sci. U.S.A.*, 78:41–45.
3. DeLeo, A. B., Jay, G., Appella, E., DuBois, G. C., Law, L. W., and Old, L. J. (1979): *Proc. Natl. Acad. Sci. U.S.A.*, 76:2420–2424.
4. Epstein, M. A., Achong, B. G., and Barr, Y. M. (1964): *Lancet*, 1:702–703.
5. Ernberg, I., Andersson-Anvret, M., Klein, G., Lundin, L., and Killander, D. (1977): *Nature*, 266:269–271.
6. Gerber, P. (1972): *Proc. Natl. Acad. Sci. U.S.A.*, 69:83–85.
7. Given, D., and Kieff, E. (1978): *J. Virol.*, 28:524–542.
8. Gurney, E. G., Harrison, R. D., and Fenno, J. (1980): *J. Virol.*, 34:752–763.
9. Hampar, B., Derge, J. G., Martos, L. M., and Walker, J. L. (1972): *Proc. Natl. Acad. Sci. USA*, 69:78–82.
10. zur Hausen, H., O'Neill, F. J., Freese, U. K., and Hecker, E. (1978): *Nature*, 272:373–375.
11. Hayward, S. D., and Kieff, E. (1977): *J. Virol.*, 23:421–429.
12. Henle, G., and Henle, W. (1966): *J. Bacteriol.*, 91:1248–1256.
13. Henle, G., Henle, W., and Diehl, V. (1968): *Proc. Natl. Acad. Sci. USA*, 59:94–101.
14. Henle, W., Henle, G., Zajac, B. A., Pearson, G., Waubke, R., and Scriba, M. (1970): *Science*, 169:188–190.
15. Hinuma, Y., Konn, M., Yamaguchi, J., Wuderski, D. J., Blekeslee, Y. R., and Grace, I. I. (1967): *Virology*, 1:1045–1051.
16. Jay, G., Khoury, G., DeLeo, A. B., Dippold, W. G., and Old, L. J. (1981): *Proc. Natl. Acad. Sci. U.S.A.*, 78:2932–2936.
17. Jörnvall, H., Luka, J., Klein, G., and Appella, E. (1982): *Proc. Natl. Acad. Sci. U.S.A.*, 79:287–291.
18. Klein, G., Clifford, P., Klein, E., and Stjernswärd, J. (1966): *Proc. Natl. Acad. Sci. U.S.A.*, 55:1628–1635.
19. Klein, G., Luka, J., and Zeuthen, J. (1980): *Cold Spring Harbor Symp. Quant. Biol.*, 44:253–261.
20. Klein, G., and Vonka, V. (1974): *J. Natl. Cancer Inst.*, 53:1645–1646.
21. Lane, D. P., and Crawford, L. V. (1979): *Nature*, 278:261–263.
22. Lindahl, T., Adams, A., Bjursell, G., Bornkamm, G. W., Kaschka-Dierich, C., and Jehn, U. (1976): *J. Mol. Biol.*, 102:511–530.
23. Linzer, D. I. H., and Levine, A. J. (1979): *Cell*, 17:43–52.
24. Linzer, D. I. H., Maltzman, W., and Levine, A. J. (1979): *Virology*, 98:308–318.

25. Luka, J., Jörnvall, H., and Klein, G. (1980): *J. Virol.*, 35:592–602.
26. Luka, J., Kallin, B., and Klein, G. (1979): *Virology*, 94:228–231.
27. Luka, J., Lindahl, T., and Klein, G. (1978): *J. Virol.*, 27:604–611.
28. Luka, J., Siegert, W., and Klein, G. (1977): *J. Virol.*, 22:1–8.
29. Matsuo, T., Hibi, N., Nishi, S., Hirai, M., and Osato, T. (1978): *Int. J. Cancer*, 22:747–752.
30. Miller, G. (1980): In: *Viral Oncology*, p. 713. Raven Press, New York.
31. Ohno, S., Luka, J., Lindahl, T., and Klein, G. (1977): *Proc. Natl. Acad. Sci. U.S.A.*, 74:1605–1609.
32. Potter, V., Witte, D. N., Coffman, R., and Baltimore, D. (1980): *J. Virol.*, 36:547–555.
33. Reedman, B. M., and Klein, G. (1973): *Int. J. Cancer*, 11:499–520.
34. Reedman, B. M., Pope, J. H., and Moss, D. J. (1972): *Int. J. Cancer*, 172–181.
35. Shapiro, I. M., Luka, J., Andersson-Anvret, M., and Klein, G. (1979): *Intervirology*, 12:19–25.
36. de Shryver, A., Freberg, S., Klein, G., Henle, W., Henle, G., de The, G., Clifford, P., and Ho, M. C. (1972): *Clin. Exp. Immunol.*, 5:443–459.
37. Strnad, B. C., Schuster, T. C., Hopkins, R. F., Heubauer, R. H., and Rabin, H. (1981): *J. Virol.*, 38:996–1004.
38. Svedmyr, E., and Jondahl, M. (1975): *Proc. Natl. Acad. Sci. U.S.A.*, 72:1622–1626.
39. Szigeti, R., Luka, J., and Klein, G. (1981): *Cell Immunol.*, 58:269–276.
40. Szigeti, R., Luka, J., Sternås, L., and Klein, G. (1982): *Int. J. Cancer*, 29:413–416.
41. Tovey, M. G., Lenoir, G., and Begon-Lours, J. (1978): *Nature*, 276:270–272.
42. Volsky, D. J., Klein, G., Volsky, B., and Shapiro, I. M. (1981): *Nature*, 293:399–401.
43. Vonka, V., Benyesh-Menich, M., and McCombs, R. J. (1976): *Int. J. Cancer*, 44:865–872.

Subject Index